BEYOND THE MAT

Don't Just Do Yoga—Live It

By Kali Om

Beyond the Mat
Don't Just Do Yoga – Live It

Author: Kali Om
Cover Design by Balogun Joy and Takao Makihara
Interior Design by Takao Makihara
Author Photo: Blair Holmes
Interior Photos: Sharon Steffensen

This book is not intended to be a substitute for the medical advice of a licensed physician. The reader should consult with their doctor in any matters relating to their physical and mental health.

Printed in the United States of America

First Printing, 2018

Print edition: ISBN 978-1-7320563-0-5
eBook edition: ISBN 978-1-7320563-1-2

Library of Congress Control Number: 2018902685

Satya Yoga and Kali Om | www.yogikaliom.com

To Sri Dharma Mittra and all spiritual preceptors

Acknowledgments

With deep gratitude to Sri Dharma Mittra, Eva Grubler Ismrittee Devi Om, Chandra Om, Devdutt Shastri, Gurudev, Carol Ann Marticke, Christian E. Jepsen, Sharon Steffensen and *Yoga Chicago* magazine, Ellen Bernstein, Takao Makihara, Mel Livatino, Miriam Marticke, my family, Burke & Grey, Richard Handler, Eric Larson, Bill Wyman, Robert Feder, Suddha Weixler, the Jois family, Lino Miele, Nancy Van Kanagan, Parvati Om, Swami Satyapremananda, Shanti Niketan Ashram, Sivananda Yoga Vedanta Centers, Cindy Lawler, Blair Holmes, Amy Krouse Rosenthal, Nathalie Martin, Amy Rome, Raghu Rama, Ralph Hannon, my teachers and students, and Hari Om.

Special thanks to the Ragdale Foundation in Lake Forest, Illinois and the Starry Night Residency Program in Truth or Consequences, New Mexico for the time, space, and vote of confidence in this work. Jai Guru!

CONTENTS

Introduction

My teachers often say that yoga is the science of living a healthy and peaceful life. Like a scientist, one takes the information, applies it, and finds out if it works. In my experience, it does; for me, yoga provides the answer to every question and the solution to every problem.

I took my first yoga class at a local YMCA shortly after my mother died of cancer, in 1997. As executor of her estate, I was not getting along with my sibling (or anyone else, for that matter), and I was racked with grief. Still, I had some time—and a lot of unstable energy after caring for her—and thought I'd give it a try.

That first class changed my life; during it I didn't think about my problems once and marveled at this new sensation. For the first time in my life, I felt real peace—and it lasted afterwards. So I signed up for every class they had.

But it wasn't enough. Consequently, I looked in the phone book and found the N.U. Yoga Center (now called the Chicago Yoga Center). I bought a monthly pass and became hooked on the physicality of Ashtanga, a traditional and challenging system from India that appealed to my past as a triathlete and pulled me right into the present. I was in class every day—sometimes twice a day, and signed up for every workshop they offered.

Within a year, one of my teachers, Eric Powell, told me he was moving away and urged me to learn how to teach and take over his classes. I refused, insisting that I was happy being a student. He asked again, and again I folded my arms and said no. The third time he asked, I said I'd think about it.

I ended up taking Suddha Weixler's teacher training at N.U. and loved it. At his request, I began teaching my own classes at his studio. More teaching opportunities soon followed. I had to quit my part-time waitressing job but continued to work as a freelance writer.

After studying with many senior Ashtanga teachers and hearing them speak about Pattabhi Jois, the father of Ashtanga yoga, I decided to "go to the source," as my mother used to say, and find out for myself. I made my first trip in 2002, not long after 9/11, when India and Pakistan were amassing their troops on the border, preparing for war. I bought an open-ended plane ticket, thinking I'd want to turn around and come home as soon as I arrived. Instead, I stayed five months, practicing with 11 other Westerners in a small, sweaty room in Pattabhi Jois's house.

I made four more trips to study with the Jois family in India, chronicling each of them in my, "No Sleep Til Mysore" diaries in *Yoga Chicago* magazine. After each trip to India, I would come home to less journalism work and more teaching gigs. I became a full-time yoga instructor in 2004, while continuing to write for *Yoga Chicago* magazine and take on other occasional writing assignments.

Pattabhi Jois used to tell us to "Think God. Be God." But it wasn't until I took my first Life of a Yogi teacher training with Sri Dharma Mittra in 2007 that I understood what he was talking about.

Although called a teacher training, it was really a course in Self-realization. It consisted of 10 intense, 15-hour days of classes at Sri Dharma's cramped old New York City studio and included instruction and practice in the complete yoga system. Each day began with chanting, *pranayama* (breathwork), and meditation, followed by talks on philosophy as well as instruction in anatomy, diet (vegetarian, mostly raw), *kriyas* (yoga techniques), Hatha yoga, *japa mala* (prayer beads), and other yoga practices. It was nothing less than a blueprint for how to live a happy and fulfilling life, and Sri Dharma's bliss, playfulness, awareness, and humility provided a living example of its efficacy. He answered all of the questions I'd never been able to articulate, all the while bombarding us with unconditional love.

Over the next several years I ended up traveling to study with him every three months and completing two more teacher trainings with him before I was kindly asked to leave the nest. Along the way, I quit taking antidepressants, received mantra initiation (and my spiritual name), and learned to love myself.

The pieces in this collection come directly from my "Beyond the Mat" column in *Yoga Chicago* magazine (2007 to 2018). Much of what I write about is derived from what I learned in the many classes, workshops, retreats, teacher trainings, and one-on-one sessions I had with Sri Dharma; from my spiritual mother, Chandra Om; from my other teachers and trainings; and from my own experience. Many of the topics were sparked by my own struggles trying to live a yogic life in a world that appears to reward exactly the opposite; the questions and concerns of my students were also an important source of material. I think of these columns as love letters—especially the more recent ones.

This collection is for anyone who wants to explore yoga in a way that goes beyond the obvious health benefits of Hatha yoga poses, or *asana*. Yoga's universal and inclusive spiritual underpinnings are often missing from mainstream American yoga instruction, when, in fact, the poses are one small part of a larger system that outlines how to live a peaceful and healthy life (and can ultimately lead to enlightenment). On the other hand, classical Raja yoga and related systems—on which I have focused my studies and writing—enable one to delve into them as deeply as one wishes (or is ready for) and be rewarded with everything from a healthy body and calm mind to Self-realization.

What I love most about what I have learned from my study of yoga is how practical and logical it is. It doesn't rely on blind faith but on direct, practical experience; the ancient yogis invited their students to try these things out for themselves, and see if they worked.

If they do, we keep them. If not, we throw them out. But this does not mean to give up if the results are not immediate. As the *Yoga Sutras* says, "practice becomes well-grounded when continued with reverent devotion and without interruption over a long period of time."

That said, everyone's path is different; what works for me may or may not work for you. I invite you to try it and find out.

What doesn't help is a closed mind. During my first trip to study with the Jois family in Mysore, I remember apologizing to Sharath Jois in one particularly rough 4:30 a.m. class for being stiff and making his attempt to provide adjustments difficult. "Body is not stiff," he said. "Mind is stiff."

After many years of giving copies of *Yoga Chicago* to students and e-mailing links to individual columns, I realized it would be more helpful to collect them in one place. For the most part, I have not altered the text of the originals; when I did, it was to ensure clarity and timeliness and to make them less Chicago-specific. Consequently, there is some overlap between the articles (in my experience, hearing things more than once helps make them stick). They're arranged loosely according to theme; my idea was not that you should read them through from start to finish (unless you want to). Rather, I hope you will choose to read columns on topics that call to you at given points in time.

I find that weaving yoga concepts into my daily life helps make it more joyful and meaningful. I hope you will too.

One of the last things Sri Dharma Mittra said to me is, "You have to share the knowledge." This is my attempt. If you find some of it helpful, it is due to the grace of God and guru. Any mistakes are on me.

Kali Om, September 16, 2017
Truth or Consequences, New Mexico

Part One: Virtues

Santosh: Cultivating Contentment

"Everything is moving perfectly."
—Sri Dharma Mittra

One of the most moving films I've seen is Jean Renoir's 1951 lyrical masterpiece, The River, based on Rumer Godden's 1946 novel. The coming-of-age tale takes place at a jute mill in pre-Independence Bengal, India. In my favorite pair of scenes, Captain John, an American soldier and former POW who lost his leg in the war, confides to Melanie, a wise Anglo-Indian teenager, that he feels like an outsider.

"I'm a stranger wherever I go," he says.

She replies quietly, "Where will you find a country of one-legged men?" She too feels like an outsider because of her mixed race.

Later, he asks Melanie what they should do. "Consent," is her answer.

"To what?" he asks.

"To everything," she says. "You don't like being a man with one leg, but you have only one leg. I don't like....never mind. Why do we quarrel with things all the time?"

Melanie's advice—to stop fighting what cannot be changed, and to make peace with one's present circumstances—is the practice of *santosh*, or contentment, which is the second *niyama* (observance) in the *Yoga Sutras of Patanjali*.

"We should understand the difference between contentment and satisfaction," explains Swami Satchidananda in his excellent 1978 commentary on the *Yoga Sutras*. "Contentment means to be just as we are without going to outside things for our happiness.

If something comes, we let it come. If not, it doesn't matter. Contentment means neither to like nor dislike."

This sounds simple on the surface. But it can require some work—especially for those of us who are used to striving or have a sense of entitlement. Here are a few concrete practices that can help.

On the mat

Many of us are guilty of destroying the present moment by wishing it away (yet all we have is the present moment; the past is gone, and the future is not guaranteed). I often see students do this in class. When they are uncomfortable or bored in a pose, they will move on to the next *asana* before the rest of us. Or they will start chugging water or looking around or staring at the mirror (some have even pulled out their phones and started using them).

There is a wonderful antidote to this feeling of discomfort in a pose (discomfort should not be confused with pain; never stay in a pose if it is causing pain and/or takes the breath away). Instead of forcing or coming out of the pose, back off about 50 percent— don't go into it as deeply—and focus on slowing down the breath. Bringing the focus back to the breath (and, if relevant, the *dristi* [gaze] and *bandhas* or locks) will almost always make it easier to stay longer in the pose. Learning how to live with discomfort (not pain!) in class, and doing poses we don't particularly like, is a form of *tapas* (self-control) that translates well to life off that mat. Coming back to the breath calms the mind and brings us back to the present moment, regardless of what we're doing.

Have you ever judged yourself in class? Perhaps you can no longer get into a pose that once came easily to you, or your body is not opening as quickly as you'd hoped (or you compare yourself to others). My first teacher, Suddha Weixler, used to regularly remind us, "It's not a competition." Learn to accept where your body is on a given day. Play with your boundaries, but never force. Find a teacher who offers variations for different bodies *and* encourages you to explore beyond your comfort zone.

Learn to become an observer, or impartial witness, of your practice. Watch your struggles with compassion, love, and patience. This practice is a type of meditation called *sakshi bhava* (witnessing mood), in which we observe our mind, body, and emotions but do not get caught up in them.

Never skip *savasana* (corpse pose), which gives us the space to spontaneously experience santosh. If thoughts bombard you—your mind keeps making plans or analyzing past events—keep bringing yourself back to the present by focusing on the sound of your breath and the sensations in your body.

Off the mat

Santosh means to detach from one's likes and dislikes, and the following practice from Swami Sivananda is very powerful: Every day, do one thing that you don't want to do and don't do one thing that you want to do. The thing you do should enhance your spiritual practice, while the one you skip can be something that derails it (for example, reading some scripture before bed and skipping the big bowl of ice cream that will make you feel awful the next day). If you have a home yoga practice, do one pose that you don't like, and skip one pose that you do.

To diminish anxiety, keep a notebook and pen next to your bed. Each morning, right after awakening, spend five minutes writing down your foremost thoughts. They can be stupid or profound or neither—it doesn't matter. The key is to write them down, which diminishes their power. I've found that when I do this, my inner critic quiets down and I feel far more content the rest of the day. This practice also helps for insomnia.

Keeping a gratitude diary for 30 days can reduce the discontent that stems from a sense of entitlement, or nonacceptance of one's circumstances. Each morning after waking, and each night before retiring, write down three things for which you are grateful, but don't repeat anything. When I did this for a few weeks, I found that I was grateful for things that normally would have bothered me. It also made me feel a whole lot more at peace. If that doesn't work, try *Karma* yoga or selfless service. Helping others who are less fortunate brings a sense of santosh very quickly.

Turn off the computer, TV, phone, and tablet for a few hours each week. Instead, spend some time in nature, or interacting face-to-face with other people, and notice the effect. (For more on detaching from electronics and slowing down, see "Do One Thing at a Time").

Understanding the laws of karma and reincarnation leads to lasting contentment. Everything we are passing through now is a result of our past actions. As my guru says, there are no accidents (or, as the *Bible* says, "Be not deceived; God is not mocked: for whatsoever a man soweth, that shall he also reap."). Although we may understand karma on a superficial level, it can take years of contemplation to realize these laws; the *Bhagavad-Gita* is the primary yoga scripture for exploring these concepts (Eknath Easwaran's translation is a good introduction). Brian Weiss's 1988 memoir *Many Lives, Many Masters* and the 2009 documentary *Unmistaken Child* are also excellent resources.

As Sri Dharma said in a 2014 interview, "This quality of contentment is derived from the realization of the laws of karma and that there is reincarnation. Also, at least for me, acceptance of the fact that: 'There is nothing else to be known or done.'"

In other words, *consent*.

Don't Hoard Your Gifts—Share Them

"It is a great opportunity if someone asks you for help. If you lose the opportunity, you may never be given another chance."
—Sri Dharma Mittra

Some years ago, I attended Mass at the church near my house, and the priest recounted the parable of the three servants.

In the story, a master gives each of his three servants a large sum of money to take care of while he takes a long trip. The two more adept servants invest their boss's money and double it. The third servant is fearful of losing the money, and buries it. When the master returns, the first two servants are commended, while the third is scolded for being lazy and wicked; the master says that he should have at least put the money in the bank, where it would have gathered interest. His money is given to the first, most adept servant. The master says, "To those who use well what they are given, even more will be given, and they will have an abundance. But from those who do nothing, even what little they have will be taken away. Now throw this useless servant into outer darkness, where there will be weeping and gnashing of teeth."

The priest explained that we must use our God-given talents, or they will be taken away.

This brought to mind a 2014 interview on the PBS news program *Chicago Tonight* with Bollywood superstar Aamir Khan, whose groundbreaking TV show, *Satyamev Jayate*, tackled formerly unspeakable issues in India—and sparked real reform. In the interview, he humbly explained that he is just trying to use his skill set—communication—to change things (and, incidentally, he was successful).

One can't help but ask....

What is your skill set?

How are you using it to help others?

There are countless examples of people who use their platforms for good, among them my guru, Sri Dharma Mittra, who has served selflessly for over 50 years. There's Oprah, John Legend, Dolly Parton, Jackie Chan, Willie Nelson, Magic Johnson, and many, many more. I'm sure you could think of a dozen on your own.

So what are *you* doing to help others? Because some yogis believe we are here for two reasons—to achieve the goal of Self-realization and to alleviate the suffering of others so that they can do the same.

Some of us find it difficult or painful to help others, especially if we have faced our own struggles in life and are still recovering from them. But that ego-driven distaste can be overcome by a strong will. The next time you see a car pulled over on the side of the road, be the first to get out and ask if you can help. Give to the homeless—especially if you don't particularly like them, or think they will spend the money on something your ego doesn't approve of (this will also help you confront any attachment to money). If you have a particular skill, share it with others, either formally (tutoring low-income students) or informally (helping an elderly neighbor navigate the Internet).

As Swami Vivekananda said, "In the world take always the position of the giver.... Give love, give help, give service, give any little thing you can....Let us give out of our own bounty, just as God gives to us."

When you help others in this way, you are practicing *Karma* yoga, the yoga of selfless action. In Karma yoga, we put our heart and soul into our work but are not attached to the outcome. Yogis believe that Karma yoga is the quickest way to surrender our identification with the ego, which separates us from our Real Self, or everlasting peace. Karma yoga is also considered a prerequisite for meditation. So if your meditation is going nowhere, start sharing your talents!

If you're reading this and scowling, remember that keeping your gifts to yourself is a form of hoarding, which is a violation of *aparigraha*, or the *yama* of nongreed. And violating yama (yoga's ethical roots) creates karma that must be accounted for down the road. So if you don't want to help others for their sake, do it for your own karma.

Hoarding your gifts can also be bad for your health, since it falls under the *guna* (quality) of *tamas*, or inertia. And according to yoga and ayurveda, all disease has its roots in tamas; first the mind becomes stuck, and then the colon–blocking toxins move into the body and make it susceptible to disease.

Tamasic behavior also keeps us stuck in old habits that prevent us from moving forward. It takes an incredible amount of energy to hold on to past patterns and beliefs—energy that could be used to help to realize our own full potential. Sharing what we have is a first step toward getting unstuck.

There are plenty of other avenues for those who are not interested in helping people, such as volunteering at an animal shelter or serving on a park cleanup crew (for other options, visit volunteermatch.org or idealist.org).

If you don't have time, give money. I still remember a *New York Times* magazine article I read long ago about college football star Michael Oher, who was a homeless teen wearing shorts and walking in the snow when Sean and Leigh Anne Tuohy took him in (their story later became the 2009 film *The Blind Side*). The reporter asked Leigh Anne why they decided to help. She said, simply, "God gives people money to see how [they're] going to handle it."

Numerous other nouns could be substituted for *money*: "God gives people talent to see how they're going to handle it," "God gives people fame to see how they're going to handle it," "God gives people healthy bodies to see how they're going to handle them," and so on.

If you don't have time or money or talent, give a smile. As Mother Teresa said, "Every time you smile at someone, it is an action of love, a gift to that person, a beautiful thing."

ॐ *Part One: Virtues*

Paring Down Can Improve Your Yoga Practice

*"A person is said to have attained to yoga when, having renounced
all material desires, he neither acts for sense gratification
nor engages in fruitive activities."*
—The *Bhagavad-Gita*

I come from a long line of pack rats. But I learned a lot about
letting go of material things during my three teacher trainings
with Dharma Mittra, especially after senior disciple Chandra Om
said that Dharma once told her she needed only two books: the
Bhagavad-Gita and the *Yoga Sutras* of Patanjali.

I'm not there yet, and perhaps I'll never be. But since then,
I've given away over three-quarters of my books (as well as half of
my clothes and shoes, not to mention most of my records, bikes,
and computers). Two apartment moves in less than a year made
it a necessity, and luckily I had the time to find a way to re-use or
recycle most of it.

Now, I live in an apartment that is relatively clean and clut-
ter-free, which makes it much easier to do my practice. After all,
one of the first instructions in the *Hatha Yoga Pradipika* is that the
space for meditation should be clean and clear.

But I still have too much stuff, and it can make the mind
anxious.

Apparently, the rest of America is also struggling with attain-
ing *aparigraha* (nongreed); the average American produces about
4.4 pounds of garbage a day, or a total of 29 pounds per week and
1,600 pounds a year, according to the Environmental Protection
Agency. According to the website A Recycling Revolution
(recycling-revolution.com), "The US population discards each
year 16,000,000,000 diapers, 1,600,000,000 pens, 2,000,000,000

razor blades, 220,000,000 car tires, and enough aluminum to re-build the US commercial air fleet four times over."

How does this happen? How do we end up buying—and wasting—so much stuff?

Some of this is due to day-to-day living. But some has to do with attachment and desire, and the inability to control the senses—ideas we are dealing with directly in yoga. By addressing these things in our daily lives, we can waste less and help the environment.

Swami Sivananda said in his "Twenty Important Spiritual Instructions": "Reduce your wants. If you have four shirts, reduce the number to three or two. Lead a happy, contented life. Avoid unnecessary worry. Be mentally detached. Have plain living and high thinking. Think of those who do not possess even one-tenth of what you have. Share with others."

Swami Narayanananda of the Sivananda Yoga Vedanta Centers brings up the Indian parable about a *saddhu* (ascetic holy person) who lives in a cave. His only possession is a loincloth. But when rats begin to eat the loincloth, he gets a cat to keep them away. The cat needs milk, so the saddhu gets a cow. The saddhu ends up spending so much time taking care of the cow, he realizes he needs to get married. In the end, he becomes a wealthy householder with many attachments.

"The idea is that wants tend to multiply themselves, so we have to be constantly on the lookout," explains Swami Narayanananda. "Swami Sivananda was always saying that we have to get rid of desires, because we know that trying to satisfy them does not work. The scriptures are very clear on it; it says very bluntly, you will never satisfy your desires. So we have to try to train ourselves in the other direction by reducing our wants, and when our mind is calling out for something and grasping for something every now and then, just denying it and practicing self-discipline. All of that helps in bringing the mind under control."

He adds that material things are not bad in and of themselves, and it's OK to live comfortably. "But if you're attached to the thing and it's your identity and reason for living, and you can't survive without it, the scriptures say you are going to suffer."

Letting go of desires is a difficult practice. But we can make a start by working on our own environment and by asking the question when making a purchase, 'Do I really need that? Do I have it already? Will I need it in such-a-such period of time?'

"Decluttering for me is like a physical manifestation of that idea," he continues. "Here [in the yoga center] it's a constant effort, because things are constantly changing. Things get cluttered up, and there's a clearing again to allow things to flow easily again, to lift the energy and increase the quality of *sattva* (peacefulness or purity)."

While decluttering our space, we can also practice the yogic idea of *ahimsa* (nonharming) with the environment in mind by recycling things or giving them to people who will use them. Chicago-based certified professional organizer Amber Kostelny says she sees more and more clients recycling or finding new homes for things, rather than just tossing them out. "Even in the kitchen, if they've overbought they'll take it to a homeless shelter or to a food pantry. I think more people are conscious of it."

But not every item can have a second life. "If you can repurpose it and let someone else use it, that's great," she says. "But it's not always the case if something is broken or missing pieces or stained. If it's not useful or you wouldn't give it to a friend or neighbor, don't give it to a charity. You see dumpsters outside of charities, because people give them stuff that isn't useful."

Amber says she sees a lot of clients who have overbought—purchased multiples of the same item—because they didn't know they already had it due to clutter. "If there are paper towels in the basement, on the first floor and the second floor, and you can't find them, you're going to go out and buy eight more rolls. I tell people to group everything in one spot, whether it's toiletries or paper towels or batteries, and to take them out as you need them. But keep them all in one spot, whatever the item may be. So then you know exactly what you have. If you don't have clutter, you don't buy the same thing over and over again," and less of it ends up in the landfill.

She says the main reasons people hold on to things is for nostalgic reasons and because "they feel like if they keep something, they could use it and they'd save money in the long run because they don't have to buy it again. And some people don't like empty spaces in their lives." There's that attachment again.

When helping clients declutter, Amber starts in the messiest area. "Just like the doctor, you want to figure out where there is the most pain, and where there is going to be the best feeling when you're done," she says.

But when doing it on your own, Amber says it's better to start in an easy area. "For some people, clothes would be easier. For another, the kitchen may be the easiest place to start; they can look at food and expiration dates very objectively: 'This is rusty, this isn't, this is expired, and this isn't.' You want to start where you can make decisions the easiest—where you're least overwhelmed." Once you've gained momentum, you can start tackling the more difficult areas.

She has a few hard-and-fast rules about decluttering: spices over a year old should be tossed. For closets, "If you didn't wear it last season, you're not going to wear it next season."

Broken items require a little more thought. "If it's going to take too much energy to fix it, don't waste the energy. I often ask, 'Is it worth your energy and time to find the missing piece or fix it?'" she says.

The hardest things to let go of are sentimental items, although the attachment usually lessens over time, which I've found to be true. "It definitely takes time to go through the grieving process, especially after the loss of a loved one," says Amber. "I see more progress with people who have let a few years go by. Then I talk through it with the clients about how to showcase these things in a way that's meaningful to them. I've seen legacy books made, I've seen people take pictures of things and frame them.

"If it's something like records or a coin collection or something really unique, it's better given to a specific outlet or organization.

"But shoving it into the back of the closet is not honoring the memory of the person or their things."

For those who are overwhelmed, there's Clutterers Anonymous (CLA), a 12-step program whose only requirement for member-ship is a desire to stop cluttering. For ideas about how to keep small living spaces free of clutter, visit apartmenttherapy.com.

When I was decluttering during my moves, I would sell things at a greatly reduced prince on craigslist.org (figuring that the buyer was paying me to remove something I no longer wanted), bring them to the Salvation Army, or find them a new home on freecycle.org.

There are also myriad books on the subject, from Michelle Passoff's *Lighten Up! Free Yourself from Clutter* to *Clutter Busting: Letting Go of What's Holding You Back* by Brooks Palmer to *The Life-Changing Magic of Tidying Up: The Japanese Art of Decluttering and Organizing* by Marie Kondo. One of my favorites is *Clear Your Clutter with Feng Shui* by Karen Kingston. Rather than buying them and having to get rid of them later, consider borrowing from the library.

If you're still stuck, try watching Anne Leonard's clever online movie, "The Story of Stuff" (storyofstuff.com). And keep in mind that having too much stuff makes it harder to do your yoga/meditation practice—if for no other reason than the eyes naturally gravitate towards clutter (and where the eyes go, the mind follows). Plus so much time is spent collecting and cleaning—or cleaning around—the stuff, you may end up shortchanging your spiritual practice. Or, worse yet, you'll run out of space for your yoga mat!

Amber says the hardest thing to do once you're organized is to maintain it. "The biggest trick to maintaining organization is putting things back where they belong."

Nowadays, I'm very careful when I go shopping. I make a list, get what I need, and leave (or at least that's what I try to do). And I regularly pass on family heirlooms to my brother and put other discards into a contractor's bag. Once it's full, I bring it to the thrift store. It's not easy, but it's worth it in order to live in peaceful surroundings.

As the *Bhagavad-Gita* says, "Which is as poison in the beginning, but is like nectar in the end; that is declared to be 'good' pleasure, born from the serenity of one's own mind."

For more tips from Amber, visit ambersorganizing.com.

4

Pratyahara: Control of the Senses

"If you control your mouth—what you put into it and what comes out of it—you've controlled much of your mind already."
—Sri Dharma Mittra

Do you eat foods that you know aren't good for you? Talk too much about useless things? Drop everything you're doing and pick up your phone the second you receive a text message alert? Eat your meals while reading, talking, or watching TV?

Then you are failing at *pratyahara*, the fifth limb of yoga, which is withdrawal or control of the senses.

Pratyahara can be a stumbling block for even the most dedicated yogi. As Sri Dharma Mittra says in his book, *Asanas: 608 Yoga Poses*, "I know many yogis in India who can renounce the world, sit under the tree, and raise their kundalini because they have no distractions. But then they come here and get tempted by the world, cars, fame, women, money, and . . . well that's why there are so many scandals around yogis. If you can overcome the temptations here, you really have mastered the senses."

Even a little bit of mastery over the senses can calm the mind, increase your energy, and improve concentration. In the *Yoga Sutras* of Patanjali, pratyahara is considered to be a bridge between the *bahiranga* (external) aspects of yoga—the first four limbs—and the *antaranga* (internal) final three limbs, which consist of concentration, meditation, and *samadhi* (divine union). And the *Bhagavad-Gita* says, "One who is able to withdraw his senses from sense objects, as the tortoise draws its limbs within the shell, is firmly fixed in perfect consciousness."

Pratyahara includes strict control of the diet. Many yogis may think their diet is under control because they have become vegan

21

or vegetarian (which corresponds to yoga's ethical injunction of *ahimsa*, or nonviolence). Yet still they overeat, or consume foods that are more tasty than healthy, such as cake, coffee, junk food, and salty snacks. Or they eat frozen, canned, processed, leftover, or convenience foods, which contain no vital energy, cause them to feel lethargic, and induce *tamas*, the quality of inertia. When choosing what to eat, it is important for the yogi to ask himself or herself: Am I feeding the senses, or am I feeding the body?

"If you are seeking enlightenment, you have to do your best to develop self-control," said Sri Dharma Mittra. "Otherwise, there will be no success in meditation (sustained concentration). You become attached to all objects of the senses. The more you enjoy the sense objects, the bigger and 'fatter' they grow."

Another important aspect of pratyahara is control of speech. In yoga, this means always speaking the truth, unless it is a harsh truth. It also means speaking only when necessary and not butting into other people's conversations or dominating conversations. Some yogis practice *mauna* (silence) for months or even years at a time.

Do you make comments on every website, or send off fiery e-mails that you later regret? Control of speech also includes other forms of communication, such as letters, voicemail, e-mail, and online commentary. A good rule of thumb is a wonderful aphorism I first encountered at the Godly Museum in Mysore, India: "Speak Less; Speak Softly; Speak Sweetly."

Yogis also control their ears—that is, they do not eavesdrop on other people's conversations (which is also considered to be a form of stealing).

Do you watch a lot of bad TV, listen to talk radio, read trashy novels, spend a lot of time on Facebook or your phone, or play a lot of video games? Would your body and mind be better served by feeding them something healthier?

When having a conversation, do you look at the other person or are your eyes darting around the room? Where your eyes go is where your *prana*, or energy, goes—and the mind follows where the prana goes. If your eyes are all over the place, then so is your mind. This includes looking around in yoga class. In Dharma yoga, we have many opportunities to practice pratyahara within the context of asana practice; closing the eyes and internalizing the focus lead to the sixth limb of yoga—concentration. In Ashtanga yoga, each pose has a *dristi* (gazing point), which serves a similar purpose.

When the senses are out of control, the energy is dissipated and the mind is not single-pointed. When the senses are under control, the energy is focused and can be directed towards whatever is important to you, whether it be your work, your family, or your spiritual practice. The *Bhagavad-Gita* says, "The man of self-control, moving among objects with his senses under restraint, and free from attachment and hate, attains serenity of mind."

Yogis believe that indulging our desires inevitably leads to more desires. As Swami Sivananda said, "Desires can never be satiated or cooled down by the enjoyment of objects. But as fire blazes forth the more when fed with butter and wood, so it grows the more when it feeds on objects of enjoyment." When we control the senses, our desires diminish and we experience *santosh* (contentment) and *sattva* (peace).

And only a sattvic mind can achieve the goal of yoga, which is Self-realization.

Even a little bit of control over the senses yields wonderful results, and makes it easier to perform one's daily tasks. But don't take my word for it. Try it for yourself.

One of the most powerful (and healthy) ways to control the senses is to clean up your diet (see "Eat Like a Yogi"). When out in public, try to avoid gossip, small talk, and idle speech. If this is hard for you, or if your mouth is always getting you in trouble, Swami Radha recommends placing a coin under the tongue, which forces you to think before you speak.

Try spending a few hours each week or an entire day in silence. This means not talking, as well as staying away from the Internet, TV, and your phone. Avoid texting in bed, and try not to check e-mail or turn on the radio first thing in the morning. Once a week or once a day, eat a meal in silence, with no distraction, and focus on what you are doing. This may cause the mind to become bored or agitated at first; try to follow through anyway.

Then, note the effect of the practice on your body and mind. Do you have more energy? Are you better able to focus? Is your mind calmer?

Only when the senses are controlled and indrawn can we experience the pure bliss that is our true nature. Yogis believe that the real treasure is inside, and we can only experience it when we stop trying to find it outside of ourselves.

5

Cultivating Gratitude and Eliminating Greed

*"The taking from anyone, including the animals and Mother
Nature without permission (or offering) is stealing. If you eat food
without being grateful, that is also a level of stealing. Learn to say,
'Thank you God, for the air I breathe. Thank you, my Lord,
to be on this planet, to have all this comfort.'"*
—Sri Dharma Mittra

A steya, or nonstealing, is the third *yama* (ethical precept) in
yoga. Many of us think, "I don't shoplift or rob banks, so I'm
good when it comes to asteya."

But like the other yamas, asteya is a deep and subtle practice that requires constant practice and unflinching self-analysis
(*svadhyaya*). It should be observed at all times, regardless of time,
place, and circumstance.

Several years ago, I was on retreat in Mexico with Sri Dharma
Mittra. A few of us decided to go to the beach one day. Afterwards,
we showered and felt great until we saw a sign that said that the
showers were for hotel guests only. We were not staying at the hotel, so we quickly found an attendant and paid for the use of the
showers.

Still think you don't violate asteya?

Do you browse the Internet for personal use while on company time? Have you ever used someone else's idea or work and not
credited them? Have you ever saved a seat or a yoga mat space for
one of your friends? Arrived late to class? Blown a stop sign when
no one was looking? Taken a towel from a hotel room?

Do you hog conversations or butt in and offer your opinion
when others are speaking? Do you live in (and heat and cool) a
house that's larger than you need, or drive short distances when

you could walk or bike? Have you ever eavesdropped or recorded someone or taken their picture without their permission? Do you overeat?

Ever file-share music and computer programs instead of paying for them? Ever fail to report income on your taxes? Arrive empty-handed for dinner at someone's home? Accumulate more yoga outfits than you need? Keep library books past their due date?

These are all violations of asteya, which, like the other yamas, is to be practiced not just in action but in speech and in thought.

Swami Sivananda said, "Taking blotting paper, pins, paper, pencil, etc. from the office is stealing. Hoarding money too much is stealing. Eating too much or gluttony is stealing. Even thinking of objects by increasing the wants is also stealing in a comprehensive sense. Keeping more things than are actually necessary is also stealing. A yoga student must be free from all these forms of theft. He must have a very clean mind—like the pure white cloth or crystal. Then alone *atman* [Self] will shine in his heart."

Some years ago, at a Navratri (Divine Mother) celebration, I jokingly pretended to walk off with the *dandas*, or sticks, we'd borrowed for a dance called the *ras garba* and immediately regretted it, as it was a violation of asteya. Indeed, even *thinking* about taking something is a violation of asteya.

The *Yoga Sutras* of Patanjali describe asteya as "noncovetousness or the ability to resist a desire for that which does not belong to us."

Another definition of asteya is to take only what is offered, and use only what is needed.

This means to stop hoarding money and objects. Imagine if we only kept what we needed, and gave away the rest to those who could use it. Life would be a lot less complicated.

Swami Sivananda said, "Why does a man steal? He wants something. When he cannot get it by legitimate ways of earning, he begins to steal things. Desire (*trsna*) or want is the root cause for stealing."

Yogis believe that desires lead to more desires; each time a desire is fulfilled, a new one appears to take its place; the cycle is endless. But once we learn to curb and control our desires, they lose their hold over us. (One way to curb desires is to wait ten days before purchasing something that is a want rather than a need; by that time, you probably will have lost interest. I like to do this with books by putting them on my wish list and then leaving them there indefinitely.)

"All of us are thieves," wrote Swami Satchidananda in his commentary on the *Yoga Sutras*. "Knowingly and unknowingly, we steal things from nature. With every minute, with each breath, we pick nature's pocket. Whose air do we breathe? It is nature's. But that doesn't mean we should stop breathing and die. Instead, we should receive each breath with reverence and use it to serve others, then we are not stealing. If we accept it and don't give anything in return, we are thieves. We steal because of greed. We want to do a little and get a lot."

So many of us live comfortable lives, yet still we think we don't have enough and keep accumulating more. If this is the case with you, consider volunteering once a week to help those who are less fortunate than you. Don't expect anything in return. You will soon realize how much you actually have. You will also start to feel a wonderful sense of purpose.

To eliminate a sense of entitlement, try beginning each meal by giving thanks to God, or nature, or everyone who helped grow the food and bring it to your plate. Consider putting aside a small portion of each meal for God (or nature, or the universe, or whatever resonates with you). Begin and end each day by giving thanks for another day of life or by reciting Swami Radha's "Divine Mother Prayer":

O Divine Mother
May all of my speech and idle talk be mantra.
All actions of my hands be mudra.
All eating and drinking be the offering of oblations unto Thee.
All lying down prostrations before Thee.
May all pleasures be as dedicating my entire self unto Thee.
May everything I do be taken as Thy worship.
Om shanti shanti shantih

Regularly take time to practice svadhyaya and contemplate your actions. How do you steal? Why do you do it? Do you feel better afterwards, or worse? Does it make your mind calm or agitated?

"Think of the evil results of stealing, namely, killing of conscience, dishonor, pin-pricks, guilty conscience, unfitness for yoga, bad name in society, punishment through the law of *karma* and penal code," said Swami Sivananda. "Think of the advantages of nontheft (asteya)—honor, clean conscience, reward in heaven, fitness for the practice of yoga. You will at once stop this stealing habit."

Ask yourself what is it that you think you are lacking that makes you feel you must take things from others. As Amrit Desai said, "The underlying premise in all stealing, coveting or jealousy is the belief that we are not sufficient, whole or complete."

But the fact is that you are sufficient, whole, and complete. The issue is that the lower nature or ego prevents your natural internal brilliance from shining forth. As Daoist master Lao Tzu said, "Be content with what you have; rejoice in the way things are. When you realize there is nothing lacking, the whole world belongs to you."

Continue to practice asteya as best you can: first in action, then in speech, and then, finally, in thought.

Rooting out one's lower tendencies is an essential step on the path of yoga. While it is difficult in the beginning, it gets easier over time.

Not only will you reap a sense of peace and contentment (*santosh*), but you will gain a special kind of wealth. The *Yoga Sutras* promises that *asteya pratisthayam sarva ratna upasthanam* ("When nonstealing is established, all jewels, or treasures, present themselves, or are available to the Yogi").

In other words, "To one established in nonstealing, all wealth comes."

6

Developing Detachment

"Detachment is not that you should own nothing,
but that nothing should own you."
—Ali ibn abi Talib

Life gives us innumerable opportunities to deal with our attachments, or the ideas, people, objects, and experiences that we cling to that don't actually belong to us. I had a wonderful opportunity to contemplate such attachments over one strange weekend a few years ago.

On Saturday, I learned that the yoga festival I was scheduled to teach at the next day had suddenly been canceled. That evening, the owner of a yoga center where I rented space for the Sunday master class I teach sent me an e-mail informing me that her studio would no longer be available to me. The following afternoon, I was driving to class on Lake Shore Drive when a police standoff closed it down. Traffic slowed down to a complete halt, and all of the alternate routes were also backed up. I finally had to realize I could not make it to class.

When I got home, I wondered if the universe was trying to tell me something. "Maybe I'm not supposed to teach yoga," I thought, and considered what life would be like without it.

Initially, the mind was agitated. But I sat with the emotions and continued to think about it. After some time, I realized it would be difficult but okay. After all, it was never my intention to become a yoga teacher (my teachers Suddha Weixler and Eric Powell convinced me to start teaching back in 1998—and over the years, and with each trip to India to study yoga, my work as a journalist diminished and my work as a teacher increased until I became a full-time yoga teacher in 2004). Through the practice of *svadhyaya* (self-study), I realized I'd had no choice when it came to becoming a yoga teacher, and that I would have no choice in how long I would continue to be one. Once I figured this out, I felt more calm. I also believe that it helped lessen my attachment to teaching yoga—at least a little bit.

The nature of attachment

In the *Yoga Sutras* of Patajani, attachment is considered to be the third *klesha*, which is described as a coloring of the mind, or a cause of pain and suffering (the other kleshas are ignorance of our divine nature, egoism, aversion, and clinging to life). Attachment is described as that which dwells in pleasure and personal preference. Yogis believe that attachments lead to pain, because pleasure is ephemeral; eventually it comes to an end—and when it does, we suffer. Yogis believe that real, permanent bliss is our true nature, which comes from inside us—not outside.

"Attachment to pleasure, or *raga*, is another pain-bearing obstacle," says Sri Swami Satchidananda in his translation of the *Yoga Sutras* of Patanjali. "We attach ourselves to pleasure because we expect happiness from it, forgetting that happiness is always in us as the true Self."

Sri Dharma Mittra asks his students to contemplate it this way. "You may notice that your happiness comes from outside: ten percent is from food; ten percent is from your spouse; and then if you have dogs, add another five percent; a nice house, add another five percent; money in the bank—it depends on the amount. If you have a job you like, add ten percent. If you have the latest iPhone, add five percent. If you like the way you look, add another 80 percent," he says.

Some of our happiness is the result of knowing that we will be able to repeat pleasurable experiences. But not forever. "Deep inside, you know that when you get old all these pleasures are going to be gone, one by one," says Sri Dharma. He says it is okay to enjoy the objects of the world while we have them—"but don't be attached." He also says that the only real, lasting happiness comes from within.

Swami Jnaneshvara (www.swamij.com) says, "Notice the moment just after pleasure: Think of times just after you experience something pleasureful. A good example is some snack food that you enjoy, such as a sweet. Notice what happens when you put a small piece of the sweet in your mouth. There is a burst of that delicious flavor, which brings an emotional joy. But then, remember what happens a second or two later. There is another emotional burst that comes right behind the enjoyment, and that is to repeat the experience. This is the meaning of attachment, or raga.... It is this *second* wave of emotional experience, or desire, that is the attachment. It is different from the enjoyment from the first piece of candy."

Ways to practice

In her memoir, *Radha: Story of a Woman's Search*, Swami Radha recalls an incident that happened at Swami Sivananda's ashram in Rishikesh in 1955. "Liz admired a gold locket I wore, which was an old family piece from my great-grandmother. It could be opened and there was a picture of Gurudev [Swami Sivananda] on the inside. Master [Sivananda] glanced up at that moment and said to me, 'Why don't you give it to her? This is the best way to renounce. If you give things to people which they greatly admire, then you will not regret that you gave them away. Renunciation is necessary to overcome attachment.'"

It's not necessary to renounce your belongings—renunciation is mental—but it is important to pay attention to what we're attached to. One way to do this is to observe what causes passion, fear, insecurity, craving, or anger; usually it comes from attachment or unfulfilled desires. Intense attachments can even become addictions. The *Bhagavad-Gita* says, "When a man dwells on objects, he feels an attachment for them. Attachment gives rise to desire, and desire breeds anger.

"From anger comes delusion; from delusion, the failure of memory; from the failure of memory, the ruin of discrimination; and from the ruin of discrimination the man perishes."

To contemplate attachment, sit for five to ten minutes in meditation and observe what the mind is attracted to. Notice what it craves. Then, do the same observation during your daily routine. "To witness this secondary process during daily life and at meditation time is an extremely useful practice to do," says Swami

Jnaneshvara. "It provides great insight into the subtler nature of *raga*, attachment. In turn, it allows a far greater level of skill in learning nonattachment, *vairagya*, which is one of the two foundation practices of yoga. By learning to witness the thinking process in this way, the colorings (klesha) gradually attenuates."

You may also take this a step further and contemplate, as I did, what it would be like to live without certain attachments. Because in reality, the things we consider to be "ours" don't really belong to us; we are merely borrowing them. The *Ashtavakra Gita* says, "One who has finally learned that it is in the nature of objects to come and go without ceasing, rests in detachment and is no longer subject to suffering."

You can also practice nonattachment with speech, substituting terms like "my" with neutral words such as "the." For example, "my car" becomes "the car," "my cat" becomes "the cat," "my house" becomes "the house," and so on. (During my first teacher training with Sri Dharma Mittra, we were encouraged not to call the students who come to our classes "my" students, since they tend to come and go and don't really belong to us.)

Another powerful practice is to let go of attachment to our pet ideas, or myths we tell ourselves about ourselves. Often these are negative, repetitive thoughts with deep roots that can be silenced through self-inquiry and discrimination.

I remember when I first began practicing yoga, and the teacher told us to try doing a handstand. I heard a familiar little voice in my head—a voice I had heard from others in the past, and which I'd internalized—telling me I was weak, and I thought, "There's no way *I* will be able to do this." But the teacher didn't know about my past, or that voice. He only saw my potential, and showed me what to do. And I did it, surprising myself, and realized that I was capable of doing much more than I'd thought.

Another very concrete way to practice vairagya, or nonattachment, is to spend some time away from the things that have a tight hold over us. For example, someone who feels attached to comfort may occasionally spend a night or two sleeping on the floor, going camping, or staying at an ashram. Someone who feels attached to their smartphone could spend several hours a week with it switched off, or leave it at home from time to time. Someone attached to TV could switch it off one night each week. Someone who feels overly attached to his or her family may choose to spend a weekend away from them. Someone who is attached to money could practice giving away a fixed amount each month, or giving a dollar or two to anyone who asks for it.

Sometimes we are attached to habits and doing the same things over and over again, and fall into a rut. One can overcome this by going outside of one's comfort zone from time to time; it can be as simple as taking a different route or form of transportation to work, or trying something new. I once waited tables with a woman who would go on what she called "fam trips" each weekend. On the "fam trip," she and her husband would visit a store, restaurant, organization, or neighborhood that they'd never been to before. She was one of the most grounded, open-minded people I've ever met.

Even just a little bit of contemplation and practice of vairagya can give you a wonderful sense of freedom and help you realize that you are much stronger than you thought you were. There will still be pain when attachments are initially ripped away, but it probably won't last long. You may also begin to see that our potential is limitless, if we would just give it a chance and take some time for self-inquiry. These realizations can lead to a deep state of *sattva*, or peace and harmony.

As the *Bhagavad-Gita* says, "The man of self-control, moving among objects with his senses under restraint, and free from attachment and hate, attains serenity of mind.

"In that serenity there is an end of all sorrow; for the intelligence of the man of serene mind soon becomes steady."

Just Say Yes: Dealing with Aversion

"Always say 'yes' to the present moment.... Surrender to what is.
Say 'yes' to life—and see how life suddenly starts working
for you rather than against you."
—Eckhart Tolle

During my first 10-day teacher training with Sri Dharma Mittra in New York City in 2007, I had to get up at 5:00 a.m. and commute for at least an hour on the F-train from Brooklyn, where I was staying, into Manhattan; spend 12 to 15 intense hours learning yoga; and then return late at night on the same train, which frequently incurred delays.

One night, after an unusually long wait on the subway platform, there was a garbled announcement saying that the F-train had stopped running; Brooklyn-bound commuters should go to another platform, take another train deeper into Manhattan, and . . . . The message trailed off. Exhausted and panicked, I wondered if I'd ever make it home. I started running down the stairs with other commuters. We stopped cold when another unintelligible announcement was made, telling us to do something completely different.

I started to run with the others and then stopped, not knowing where to go. At that moment, I realized that I could spend the night on the train if necessary, and it would be OK. Relieved, I took a breath and looked around. The woman next to me caught my eye and asked where I was headed. "Park Slope," I said. "Me too," she replied, smiling. "Let's share a cab."

Sometimes, when we accept a situation, it solves itself.

Indeed, much of our pain and suffering comes from having expectations about the way we think things will be, and they turn out differently (e.g., we plan a picnic and it rains). Instead of dealing with the situation, we resist it. When we do this, the mind often adds some old memories and starts churning out of control and putting us into what Eckhart Tolle in his 2005 book, *A New Earth: Awakening to Your Life's Purpose*, calls "the pain body." Next thing you know, we're miserable and taking everything personally.

"Why sometimes does life become so difficult?" asks Swami Vishnudevananda in his 2015 book, *Teachings on Yoga Life*. "What is the real difficulty? I will tell you. The difficulty is only in our mind. There are no difficulties. Many of us fight against the natural flow of life whether consciously, or even subconsciously, without knowing that we are struggling. But if we do this, our energy, our *prana* [vital life force], is eaten away by the fight. Others among us manage challenges easily because we may have already experienced enough difficulties in our lives to have come to an understanding that resistance brings suffering. Each one of us, teacher and student alike, has to eliminate the negativity in the mind, because otherwise it stays with us throughout our lifetime, and we lead an unfulfilled life. When the opportunity arises to rid ourselves of negativity, we have the choice to surrender or to resist. To change by surrendering is not easy; it is like being burnt. Remember though, that once that moment of pain has gone, it has gone forever and we emerge stronger."

In other words, surrendering can initially be painful and even feel a little frightening. But fighting the way things are causes more pain, not to mention a great loss of energy. When we try to rush or control things, we fall out of the natural flow of life. This causes us to feel more separate from others, which thickens the ego (*asmita*, or egoism, is the second *klesha*, or cause of pain and suffering, on the path of yoga) and makes us feel like we're swimming upstream. Our consciousness and world contract, and we live in anger and fear. In other words, resistance, or *dvesha* (aversion, the fourth klesha), only increases our suffering and makes us feel like the world is a hostile place.

When we accept what we cannot change and go with the flow—even if it's initially difficult—the ego begins to thin. We feel open to life; we feel taken care of, and our consciousness expands. Fear is replaced by trust, and we start to feel surrounded by love.

We have an invitation to do this in every moment. Wonderful things are happening around us all the time if we'd just stop resisting what is, and pause to notice them. Tolle calls it coming into presence. "When you recognize that the present moment is always already the case and therefore inevitable, you can bring an uncompromising inner 'yes' to it and so not only create no future unhappiness, but with inner resistance gone, find yourself empowered by Life itself," he writes in *A New Earth*. This means sitting with the situation and any emotions it brings up, rather than fighting them.

Being in the present is sometimes referred to as flow. "It is when we act freely, for the sake of the action itself rather than for ulterior motives, that we learn to become more than what we were," writes Mihaly Csikszentmihalyi in his seminal 2008 book, *Flow: The Psychology of Optimal Experience*. "It is by being fully involved with every detail of our lives, whether good or bad, that we find happiness, not by trying to look for it directly."

"I think there's a lot of similarity between what people try to do with religion and what they want from art," musician Brian Eno once said. "In fact, I very specifically think that they are the same thing. Not that religion and art are the same, but that they both tap into the same need we have for surrender."

Surrender to the will of the divine, or *ishvara* (also *isvara*) *pranidhana*, is the fifth niyama (observance) in *Raja* (royal) yoga; it means constantly living with an awareness of one's own true nature and surrendering to the will of the universe.

"Isvara pranidhana, or devotion to the all-knowing Isvara, is another method for obtaining Samadhi," says Swami Satchidananda. "It is the emotional path which is easier than other methods. . . just surrender yourself unto Him, saying, 'I am Thine; all is Thine; Thy will be done.' The minute you have resigned yourself completely, you have transcended your ego."

Surrender means to trust that life is unfolding exactly as it should be. A direct and practical way to surrender when things are difficult is to look at past problems and realize that things have always turned out for the best. (If they hadn't, you wouldn't be reading this.)

Chandra Om once said, "Walking by faith means being prepared to trust where we are not yet permitted to see. This kind of

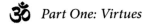

faith knows nothing of doubt, discouragement, or impossibilities, but solely in success and trust in God."

Someone close to the Dalai Lama was once asked what he is like in person. "The smallest person in the room," he replied. In other words, he has no agenda; there is no craving and no seeking or sense of entitlement. Just presence.

"We expect there to be some sort of prize, some sort of gift for us in the world out there," writes Tony Parsons in his 2003 book, *All There Is*. "All the time we are looking for that, we are not seeing what is already there. Awakening is simply the dropping of looking for something. It's the dropping of the one that seeks. That's all it is.

"And once that acceptance is there, there is also an acceptance of the character, the character in the play, the 'me.' There is an acceptance of this body/mind organism that walks around on this stage. It is simply seen and taken in, in love. Once there is an acceptance of this character, then there is an acceptance of all the other apparent characters. It is seen that this is simply all the one manifesting.

"This is really what unconditional love is."

The Practice of Satya (Truthfulness)

"Always speak the truth—but never a harsh truth."
—Swami Brahmananda

I can't count how many times students have said to me, "See you in class tomorrow!" and failed to show the next day.

This is a breach of *satya*, or truthfulness. Satya is one of the five *yamas*, or ethical roots of yoga: nonharming, nonstealing, continence, nongreed, and truthfulness. According to the *Yoga Sutras* of Patanjali, the yamas are to be practiced in word, thought, and deed—regardless of time, place, and circumstance.

Satya means communicating honestly and following through on our obligations and commitments, even if it's no longer convenient. Like the other yamas, satya can be a practice in and of itself. It goes far beyond simply telling the truth when asked a question (such as, "Did you cut down the cherry tree?").

Not following through on one's word about coming to class doesn't hurt the teacher, who will be there anyway. But it does hurt the student who has lied to herself (a violation of *ahimsa*, or nonharming). Yogis believe that each time we violate one of the yamas, it is like we are breaking our own heart; each instance blocks the peace and tranquility we are seeking through yoga. According to my guru, Sri Dharma Mittra, on a subtle level, this can block the *nadis* (energy channels in the subtle body), making our inner light shine a little less brightly.

In the book *Sivananda's Gospel of Divine Life*, there's a wonderful story about Swami Sivananda instructing his disciples.

"While the Master was leaving the bhajan hall after the satsang was over, a visitor approached him and requested he be allotted some time for an interview.

"'Five o'clock tomorrow, but no promise,' replied the Master.

"Then, turning to the people around him, [Swami Sivananda] said, 'Do not give any promise. Even if you are sure of going to a certain place at 10 a.m., do not say, "I will go." Say, "I will try." This is my method. Otherwise, if you fail to go, people will say that you had promised and did not fulfill it.'"

Satya means being sincere. Exaggeration, bragging, and gossiping are considered breaches of satya. Padding one's résumé or bio, inflating one's experiences, and taking credit for someone else's work (or not giving them credit) all fall into this category. So does being a hypocrite, such as telling others how to act and not trying one's best to follow the same injunction, or pretending to be something one is not.

Truthfulness can be practiced on the mat in yoga class by being self-aware. If you are a beginner, it is important to practice at a beginning level, rather than trying the advanced variations before you are ready (and inviting injury). Similarly, more seasoned students should do their best to work intelligently at their level.

Satya also means reporting our income truthfully on our tax returns, regardless of how we feel about paying taxes and the federal government. "If you are paying the taxes and doing everything according to the laws, you feel secure and happier," says Sri Dharma Mittra.

Satya can be practiced first in small ways. If you make a mistake, it's best to own up to it (without delay) rather than hiding or letting someone else take the blame. Another way is to speak truthfully in a confident, straightforward manner. Do not mumble, mince words, or be a "low talker." If someone invites you to an event that you're not sure you want to attend, say "Let me get back to you." Then politely decline, via e-mail if necessary. But do not procrastinate on giving your answer. Avoid saying "I'm sorry" unless you mean it and it's warranted.

Ideally, one should tell the truth at all times—unless it hurts someone. Then, nonviolence, or ahimsa, takes precedence. *Manu Smriti* (an ancient Hindu legal text) says, "One should speak what is true; one should speak what is pleasant; one should not speak what is true if it is not pleasant, nor what is pleasant if it is false. This is the ancient dharma."

Sometimes, though, you have to say *no* in order to be truthful, because saying "no" to someone else can sometimes mean saying "yes" to yourself. (This can be especially true when it comes to *sadhana*, or spiritual practice.) In other words, don't break the promises you have made to yourself.

Satya also means following your inner intuition. If something feels wrong, or goes against your conscience, do you continue to do it anyway because of outside pressure or because it's convenient? On her radio show, Dr. Laura Schlessinger once cited a study of women who had serious misgivings about their marriage partners as they stood at the altar. Yet all of them went through with their weddings. And all of them ended up divorced!

Swami Radha said, "If there is a conflict between the life that you are living and the one you should be living, your inner conflict will grow and grow and grow. Then the Divine will say, 'That's enough now. I have given you a lot of rope. You have tried all things that everybody else is doing. That's finished now.' And then something dramatic or painful may come into your life to make you change."

When we are established in satya, the mind becomes calm. We have fewer worries and are less likely to wake up in the middle of the night with our thoughts spinning out of control. We are able to tune in to the quiet, still voice within, and our meditation improves.

Swami Sivananda said, "God is truth, and He can be realized by observing truth in thought, word and deed." According to him, the 13 forms of truth include: truthfulness, equality, self-control, absence of jealousy, absence of envious emulation, forgiveness, modesty, endurance, charity, thoughtfulness, disinterested philanthropy, self-possession, and unceasing and compassionate harmlessness.

Speaking the truth gives you tremendous willpower. The *Yoga Sutras* states that when our words match our actions and our convictions—when we are perfectly established in satya—what we say becomes true.

The first step toward becoming established in satya is to be aware of when we violate it, and note it in your spiritual diary (see "Keep a Spiritual Diary"). Swami Sivananda advises, "Acknowledge your faults openly and endeavor to rectify yourself in the future." In other words, learn from your mistakes, but don't beat yourself up about them. Start fresh the next day with more awareness and firm resolve not to repeat them.

Satya is not an easy practice. But as Swami Vivekananda said, "Comfort is no test of truth. Truth is often far from being comfortable."

Part Two: The Seasons

ॐ *Part Two: The Seasons*

The 30-Day Resolution

"Practice alone brings success."
—The *Hatha Yoga Pradipika*

I read that during his *sadhana* (period of spiritual practice), Swami Sivananda practiced one virtue for 30 days, and, once it was established, moved on to another one.

"His method of developing a virtue was to take one at a time and practice it for a month," writes Swami Sahajananda in *Sivananda's Gospel of Divine Life.*

I was immediately reminded of the 30-day plans we followed during Sri Dharma Mittra's 500-hour Life of a Yogi teacher training. In 2008 I was among a group that spent four-day weekends once a month for four months studying directly with Sri Dharma at his New York center. At the end of each session, we were given very specific 30-day plans to follow at home, which included *asana* (poses), *pranayama* (breathing practices), concentration, meditation, and diet practices, and we signed them in front of Sri Dharma. We were also required to record our experiences in a spiritual diary. These 30-day practices resulted in rapid spiritual progress—and were easy to continue after the 30 days ended.

This year, rather than making an annual resolution that usually results in failure, consider making a dozen 30-day plans or resolutions (you can come up with new plans each month, or expand upon a previous one). They can be for something as simple as meditating or doing pranayama for five minutes a day, going to yoga class three times a week, or whatever you think would strengthen your spiritual practice.

Just make sure you choose one thing to work on at a time, or you are likely to fail. And be very specific. As consultant and author

Tony Schwartz wrote in a 2015 *New York Times* op-ed piece, "We humans have a very limited reservoir of will and discipline. We're far more likely to succeed by trying to change one behavior at a time, ideally at the same time each day, so that it becomes a habit, requiring less and less energy to sustain."

Practice
There are many places to start; if cleaning up your apartment or fixing your finances will help your spiritual practice, vow to work on it for 10 minutes a day. If you want to improve your *hanumanasana* (splits), do the same thing.

If you want to accelerate your spiritual practice in a more direct way, here are a few places you could start:

Gratitude
A few years ago, I heard local longtime Chicago *yogini* Radha (Gloria McCartney) discuss her daily gratitude practice and decided to give it a try for 30 days. Each morning after waking, and each night before retiring, I wrote down three things for which I was grateful; the catch was that I could not repeat anything. After a few days, all latent anger and anxiety dissipated. After a couple of weeks, I found myself writing down things that normally would have bothered me ("angry woman in alley") and saw how they were helping me. By the end of the month, I had cultivated more mindfulness and *santosh* (contentment, or being at peace with the here and now). It's an incredibly powerful practice.

Ahimsa (nonharming)
All of the other yogic virtues come from compassion, or ahimsa, toward all living beings. To practice ahimsa toward animals, consider giving up meat for a month. If that's too much, consider giving it up once or twice a week, and notice the results. Or simply try not to hurt others (even the people you don't like) in action, speech, or thought. Doing *Karma* yoga (selfless service, or helping others who are less fortunate) can help increase one's compassion.

Satya (truthfulness)
Focus on talking less and speaking only the truth (for example, don't make promises you're not going to keep). If you say you're coming to class, come to class. If you're not sure, say "I will try."

Asteya (nonstealing) and aparigraha (nongreed)
Take or use a little bit less than you need, whether it's food or energy or something else. For example, turn off the lights when you're not using them, and turn down the heat when you're not home. Consider carpooling or riding your bike when possible. If you're not using something (and not planning to use it), give it away to someone who will. If you are always late, work on punctuality for a month, since wasting other people's time is a form of stealing. Give thanks before you eat (on a subtle level, *not* giving thanks is also considered a form of stealing).

Pratyahara (control of the senses)
Pratyahara can be practiced in countless ways, including everything from limiting the amount of junk food you consume to staying off the Internet and/or phone for an hour or two a day (or week) to using *dristis* (gazing points) during your yoga practice.

Svadhayaya (self-study)
Read or study scripture for a few minutes each day (this is lovely to do right before bed), and contemplate what you've learned. Keep a spiritual diary.

Pranayama (breathing practices)
If you're not used to pranayama, start with something simple and easy such as deep diaphragmatic breathing for five or 10 minutes a day. If you have an existing practice, vow to do it daily for 10 minutes or more. Ideally, try to practice at the same time each day.

Dharana/dhyana (concentration/meditation)
If you already have a sitting meditation practice, vow to do it daily for five to 30 minutes. If not, try focusing on the breath or concentrating at *trikuti* (the third eye), which can help dispel depression and stimulate inner intuition. Or meditate for 10 minutes a day on

one of Swami Sivananda's 12 virtues outlined in *How to Cultivate Virtues and Eradicate Vices:*
Humility in January
Frankness (*arjava*) in February
Courage in March
Patience in April
Mercy (*karuna*) in May
Magnanimity in June
Sincerity in July
Pure love in August
Generosity in September
Forgiveness in October
Balanced state in November
Contentment in December

Conclusion

Choose one thing to work on for the first month, then see if you can come up with a plan for the other 11 months of the year so you have a road map. Be as specific as you can ("10 minutes of such-and-such pranayama every day at 8 a.m."). Write down your plan, sign it, and give it to someone you trust (or burn it). Work on it for a month, and then move on to the next practice (the first practice may have become a habit by then). Check it off each day you practice, and note any experiences you have in your spiritual diary. Notice when you fail, but don't beat yourself up about it. Instead, vow to start fresh the next day.

You will find that you start to transform yourself, little by little. Because that's what yoga ultimately is: self-transformation, or a slow diminishing of one's lower nature into one's highest self, or *satchidananda* (pure existence, consciousness, and bliss).

But don't put it off until next year. As Swami Sivananda said, "D.I.N.!" (Do it now!)

Beat the Winter Blues

"Like the seeds dreaming beneath the snow
your heart dreams of spring."
—Kahlil Gibran

I used to be a lethargic depressive.

You know—the kind who never has any energy and doesn't want to get out of bed. The type who only wants sleep and eat, and eat and sleep, who doesn't even want to see her friends, and for whom even the smallest task seems insurmountable.

This is how many otherwise cheerful people feel during the winter months, if they suffer from seasonal affective disorder (SAD). SAD symptoms can include decreased energy and concentration, a lack of interest in work and social activities, increased appetite (especially for carbohydrates), increased sleep, social withdrawal, and feelings of hopelessness. While most people experience a shift to lower energy levels in winter, SAD sufferers experience classic symptoms of depression.

I started getting my depression under control in 1997, about a month after my mother died of cancer. That's when I walked into my first yoga session at the local YMCA. The class provided a vacation from the ever-present pain, and the sense of well-being lasted for a few hours afterwards. I was hooked from the start. Within a few months, I was taking classes every day (sometimes twice a day) at the Chicago Yoga Center; a year later, at my teachers' urging, I was sharing what I'd learned with others.

Since then, I've devoted my life to the study and practice of yoga, studying with a long list of senior instructors, making five trips to India, completing over ten teacher trainings, and continuing my practice and studies. I have been able to fine-tune my practice to the point where I could throw out my antidepressants.

I still struggle with mood swings. But now, I have a yoga arsenal at my disposal.

Now, I can alter my mood using postures, breathing, mudras, diet, chanting, and meditation. Here are a few things that may help you.

Move

Backbends and twists are great for combating lethargy, because they affect the spine and activate the nervous system, releasing energy. Supported backbends are a wonderful option if you're feeling depleted; it can be as simple as lying down with a bolster supporting your middle back, and placing a rolled blanket under the shoulders.

But I've found that simply moving the body will make the energy start to flow. If you haven't yet developed a home yoga practice, get yourself to class! (If you find classes too expensive, find out if your local studio has a free community class, or check the offerings at the local park district.) Or simply go outside and take a brisk walk around the block. Just make sure you do it when the sun is out, so you can soak up its energizing rays.

Breathe

The breath contains *prana*, or the vital life source. It follows that if you breathe deeply, you'll bring more prana into the body and feel less lethargic. When I'm feeling depleted, I do a positive breathing exercise I learned from Sri Dharma Mittra. I combat anxiety with calming breathing. These practices—and most *pranayamas* (breathing techniques)—should be learned directly from a qualified teacher.

A type of breathing that requires no special training is smooth, even diaphragmatic breathing through the nose. You may do this breathing anywhere, at any time. Initially, try it on your back, while in *savasana* (final resting pose), placing your hands on the belly and chest and noticing the movement of the breath. Make sure the inhale is as long as the exhale and that the belly is moving. Adding *ujjayi*, or victorious breath, by making a gentle snoring or hissing sound in the back of the throat draws the mind's attention to the breath and automatically has a calming effect. As the *Chandogya Upanishad* says, "He who has control of his breath also has control over his mind."

Chant

There's a reason that the Hare Krishnas sell a book called *Chant and Be Happy*—it works. The ancient yogis discovered that sound vibrations have a profound effect on the mind, and there is a *mantra* (repeated sound) for every situation. The simplest mantra of course is "Om" (or "Aum"). The first part, "A," is pronounced with an open mouth, as in "father." The second sound is "o," as in "home," with an O-shaped mouth. The third part is "m," which is pronounced with the lips together. After chanting Om, sit still for a moment and feel the vibration. Then start again. You may do this for several minutes. Om is considered an *anahata nada*, or an unstruck sound. The *Katha Upanishad* states that Om is "the best support; this is the highest support. Whosoever knows this support is adored in the world of Brahma." Whether you believe this or not, the sound creates a gentle, soothing vibration that stimulates the pituitary gland and restores a sense of well-being.

If you are not inclined to chant, I've found that simply opening the mouth and singing along to a favorite song can also have a positive effect.

Read

Sri Dharma Mittra says, "When you become depressed, it is because you are neglecting your spiritual practice." When I'm feeling off-kilter, reading from the *Bhagavad-Gita* or the *Yoga Sutras* usually puts me right back on track. If you come from another spiritual tradition, open one of your holy books to any page, read a few paragraphs, and reflect on it. If you don't have a spiritual tradition, use any book that inspires and uplifts you, such as poetry or philosophy or a favorite work of fiction. If you don't like to read, look at an inspiring piece of art, or listen to a favorite piece of music. I like to do this right before bed, to set a positive tone for the next day.

Relax

Sri Dharma Mittra calls relaxation the greatest antidote to impurities. When you feel too tired to get up and move, try taking a long savasana. Light a candle or incense. Turn down the lights, or cover your eyes. Lie on your back with the palms facing up near the hips, and the feet falling out to the sides. Systematically, release every muscle in the body, starting with the feet and moving up to the crown of the head. (If you find this difficult, I recommend listening to Chandra Om's excellent *Yoga Nidra* recording.) Remain in savasana for at least 12 minutes, which master yoga teacher Judith Lasater says is the minimum needed to induce a state of deep relaxation. Sometimes, taking time for relaxation can heal the body and mind like nothing else in the world. And if you fall asleep, well, it's probably because you're not getting enough sleep!

Mahashivaratri: The Great Night of Lord Shiva

"The entire universe, animate and inanimate, comes from me.
Everything is seen through me. Everything comes to rest in me.
I am no different from it and nothing in this world is different from me."
—The *Shiva Samhita*

I first learned about Maha Shivaratri in 2002, when I was in Mysore, India, studying Ashtanga Vinyasa yoga with Pattabhi Jois. There were no classes that day or the next because he was fasting all day and keeping vigil all night, chanting the name of Lord Shiva—the ideal yogi, often portrayed sitting in meditation on Mt. Kailash, who represents the Supreme Self.

That night I sat on the roof of the lodge where I was staying, eating pizza with another student who was returning home to England the next day. First, we gazed west and watched the sunset. Then we turned our plastic chairs toward the east and looked toward the Mysore Palace, where there was an all-night *puja* (ritual worship) in Lord Shiva's honor. Suddenly, the palace lights came on, brightening the evening sky.

Six years later, during a training with Sri Dharma Mittra, I learned from one of the teachers that Maha Shivaratri, also called just Shivaratri, is the most important night of the year for yogis and that every time one chants "Om Namah Shivaya" that night, it has the power of chanting it 1,000 times. ("Om Namah Shivaya," known as the great five-syllable mantra, means prostrations to Lord Shiva. Its syllables—Na, Ma, Shi, Va, and Ya—symbolize the five elements: earth, water, fire, air, and *akasha*, or ether.)

Shivaratri celebrates the night that Lord Shiva married the goddess Parvati; it falls on the new moon day in the month of Maagha in the Hindu calendar (usually February or March; a quick online search will reveal the current year's date). Often, you can find all-night vigils held at Hindu temples and at places such as a Sivananda Yoga Vedanta Center.

It also celebrates the night when Lord Shiva performed the *tandava*, the cosmic dance of destruction symbolized by *natarajasana* (lord of the dance pose). According to another legend, Shiva saved the world from the poison that emerged during the churning of the sea by consuming it and used his yogic powers to hold it in his throat, which is why his neck is blue and he is called *Neela Kantha*, or the Blue Throated (which is among the 108 names of Lord Shiva that are often chanted on Shivaratri).

Lord Shiva, the father of Ganesh and Subramanya, is considered to be the supreme lord of the yogis, who is simultaneously a householder and a celibate renunciate. According to the website of author and yoga scholar David Frawley (Pandit Vamadeva Shastri), Lord Shiva is "the great ascetic and yogi, reflecting the highest self-discipline and inner equipoise. He indicates the power that pervades the universe and allows us to ascend in consciousness to our highest potential, which is that of Self-realization" (vedanet.com).

Frawley continues, "Yoga as a *sadhana* or spiritual practice rests upon cultivating the Shiva consciousness of the highest awareness and bliss. This reality of Shiva is the power of silence, stillness, and non-doing, not the ordinary power of self-assertion and aggression. It works through inaction, peace and balance, in which one is centered in one's own being and grasps the entire universe as a manifestation of one's own thoughts. This power of Shiva is not the outer force that displays itself for personal gain, nor the outer effort to control that makes a show of itself to gain adulation. It is the spiritual force that turns things around, draws things within, and takes them back to their source, in which a deep unity remains. Shiva symbolizes this balancing and calming effect of all Yoga practices."

The year after I learned about the importance Maha Shivaratri, I celebrated by myself in my poorly heated apartment, fasting all day and chanting "Om Namah Sivaya" until I couldn't take the cold any longer and went to sleep. The following year, the swami from the Sivananda Yoga Vedanta Center invited me to come to their all-night puja and *kirtan* (chanting); it was wonderfully energizing and inclusive, but I had to leave at 1 a.m. The following year I was able to stay the whole time, after which I taught two 90-minute yoga classes in a row (I was so spiritually charged that I could have taught more; instead I went home and took a nap). Since then, I've made it through the entire puja each year and have even led some chants and was once the assistant *pujari* (performer of the puja). Fortunately, it is auspicious to attend even a small part of Shivaratri.

In addition to fasting, keeping vigil, and singing hymns on Shivaratri, according to Swami Sivananda, the *lingam* (a phallus representative of the eternal, still Shiva or pure awareness) "is worshipped throughout the night by washing it every three hours with milk, curd, honey, rose water, etc., whilst chanting the mantra 'Om Namah Shivaya.' He who utters the names of Shiva during Shivaratri, with perfect devotion and concentration, is freed from all sins. He reaches the abode of Shiva and lives there happily. He is liberated from the wheel of births and deaths."

Frawley writes, "Shiva is the great guide to meditation, the supreme guru, teaching us to observe, contemplate and not react, providing us with a cosmic view of the events in our lives and the emotions in our minds, so these can never overwhelm us. Yet Shiva is not the deity of a mere intellectual meditation or any mere personal self-analysis; he is the deity of merging the mind back into its source in the infinite, giving up the personal mind for the universal consciousness. Shiva takes us beyond the preconceptions of the mind to the consciousness that pervades all space and is not bound to any memory patterns, fears or desires."

Symbolism in the portrayal of Lord Shiva
- Trident (*trishula*) represents the three states (waking, dreaming, and deep dreamless sleep) and the three *gunas* or qualities of nature (*sattva* [harmony or wisdom], *rajas* [energy or passion], and *tamas* [inertia, inaction, or darkness]) and shows that Lord Shiva is beyond them
  - Third eye (*trikuti*) represents divine perception or wisdom
  - Matted hair (*jata*) represents Shiva as being beyond the standard definitions of beauty and holiness

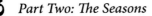

- Crescent moon in hair represents mastery over time
- Ganges in hair represents the flow of spiritual knowledge symbolized by the holy river
- Serpent around neck represents mastery of the ego and Shiva as beyond the powers of death
- Drum (*damaru*) represents creation and Om, from which all languages are formed
- Tiger skin represents control of lust
- Blue neck represents suppression of evil (Shiva consumed poison to save the world from destruction)
- Ashes on body represent the temporary nature of the body

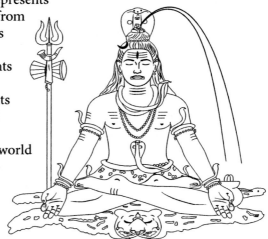

Internal Spring Cleaning

"Be kind to everyone; forgive everyone everything."
—Sri Dharma Mittra

Spring is a new beginning and an ideal time to let go of what's holding us back.

In one season opener of the TV series, *Yogi Cameron: A Model Guru*, ayurvedic therapist Yogi Cameron (YC) treats a 25-year-old with autism named Zach. Zach is angry, and YC wants to know why. Zach says other children at the synagogue he attended harassed him. "How old were you when that happened?" YC asked. "Seven or eight," Zach replied. "That was a long time ago," says YC. "When are you going to let it go?"

In modern American culture, we tend to hold on to grievances from times long past and use them as an excuse to avoid dealing with the things we don't like about our life: I'm not living up to my potential because my parents beat me / spoiled me / weren't there for me / were too strict with me / gave me too much freedom or attention / ignored me / favored my siblings over me / [your excuse here]. In America, we like to play the blame game and say that our problems are someone else's fault.

But in yoga we understand that the soul is eternal, and that our soul, or *atman*, chooses the parents we will have and the circumstances we find ourselves in. In yoga, we know that these birth families or circumstances give us the best possible opportunity to burn off our old *karma* (spiritual principle of cause and effect) and learn the lessons we need to know in this lifetime—that each unpleasant thing is happening for a reason, according to our deeds from the past.

I first heard about the laws of karma and reincarnation in the 1970s, when the film, *The Reincarnation of Peter Proud,* aired on TV. But I didn't really believe in it until 30 years later, when I heard about it from the lips of my guru, Sri Dharma Mittra, and realized that everything we are going through now is a result of our past deeds. He shared his own experiences and backed them up with passages from the great yoga scripture the *Bhagavad-Gita.* When I thought about what he said, I realized that everything "bad" that happened to me in my life—and believe me, there was a lot of unpleasantness—led to something good. Every single time. I realized that these "bad" experiences taught me a lesson, fostered personal growth, or set my life in a new direction (such as when my mother died and I started practicing yoga), and I stopped taking them personally.

As the *Bhagavad-Gita* says, "That which is like poison at first but like nectar in the end—that happiness, born of the clear knowledge of the Self, is said to be of the nature of sattva [peace and harmony]." Sri Dharma often says he is thankful when something unpleasant happens to him, because it means he has burned off one more karma.

This is easy to understand on an intellectual level. Yet many of us still have doubts and see ourselves flogging the same old dead horse, over and over, stuck in our old ways of being, thinking, and acting. If we do this long enough, we could end up with a terrible illness. Because in yoga, it is believed that all disease begins in the mind.

So, this spring, give it some thought: Is there something you haven't let go of that is holding you back? Is there someone you need to forgive, or someone of whom you should ask forgiveness? (Mahatma Gandhi said, "The weak can never forgive. Forgiveness is the attribute of the strong.")

Is there someone you need to thank? Is there someone you need to confront, or to cut loose from because the relationship is no longer serving you? Do you need to forgive yourself for something?

What is holding you back from doing what you want with your life?

It is never too late to ask these questions, and though it can be done anytime, spring is a wonderful time of year to let go, an opportunity to begin anew. The most direct way is to do this internally, by practicing *svadhyaya*, or self-study. This can be done in meditation and through journaling, by asking and answering the questions posed above.

Svadhyaya can be helped by the physical act of letting things go and clearing out the clutter in your living space. Because if there's clutter at home, there is clutter in the mind. Perhaps it is your stuff—mental, physical, spiritual—that is holding you back.

Often, when we make an external effort, what we need to do internally becomes abundantly clear. After all, cleaning and organizing is a type of meditation (and spring is the best time to do it; see "Paring Down Can Improve Your Yoga Practice"). Another wonderful resource for getting started is Karen Kingston's 1999 book *Clear Your Clutter with Feng Shui: Free Yourself From Physical, Mental, Emotional and Spiritual Clutter Forever.*

Once the physical debris is out of the way, it is much easier to work on internal letting go.

There are many ways to express forgiveness. It can be done in person, or on the phone, or in a letter (I do not recommend doing it via e-mail, voicemail, Facebook, or texting, which would smack of insincerity). It can also be done mentally, if the person is no longer around or still poses a threat to you. (There is no need to stir up trouble or reopen old wounds; in some cases it is best to let sleeping dogs lie, and offer forgiveness mentally. Sri Dharma always says, "Love the bad man, but keep the distance.")

Sometimes, we come to realize that we have caused harm and need to ask forgiveness, which can be done in much the same way. Just keep it simple and straightforward, name exactly what you are sorry for, express your regret at causing harm, and do not make excuses for your behavior.

There are many types of forgiveness meditation. One of the most simple and direct is from former Buddhist monk and author Jack Kornfield. As with any meditation, begin by sitting comfortably in a quiet place where you will not be disturbed (if the floor is not comfortable, sit in a chair with the head, neck, and spine in a straight line). Breathe deeply and comfortably, and contemplate how forgiveness can help you soften your heart.

Begin by asking forgiveness of others you have harmed. Visualize each situation where you have caused pain, and experience the emotions it elicits. Realize that you only caused them harm because of your own pain, fear, anger, or confusion. Then, say to each person, "I ask for your forgiveness, I ask for your forgiveness."

Next, focus on forgiving yourself for all of the times you have wittingly or unwittingly been the cause of your own pain. Visualize each instance and feel the emotions. Then, say to yourself, "For the ways I have hurt myself through action or inaction, out of fear, pain, and confusion, I now extend a full and heartfelt forgiveness. I forgive myself, I forgive myself."

Finally, focus on forgiving those who have harmed you. Imagine each episode, and allow the emotions to come up. Then, repeat the following: "I now remember the many ways others have hurt or harmed me, wounded me, out of fear, pain, confusion, and anger. I have carried this pain in my heart too long. To the extent that I am ready, I offer them forgiveness. To those who have caused me harm, I offer my forgiveness, I forgive you."

Don't be surprised if this practice is difficult at first. It can take a lot of time to master it. You may find it helpful to start with small things, and work towards bigger ones.

As Kornfield said, "Forgiveness cannot be forced; it cannot be artificial. Simply continue the practice and let the words and images work gradually in their own way. In time you can make the forgiveness meditation a regular part of your life, letting go of the past and opening your heart to each new moment with a wise loving kindness."

You may find you prefer a different forgiveness meditation. Or you may create your own; it is important that the practice feel authentic to you. That way you're more likely to actually do it, and your efforts will be unforced.

Just remember that any sincere effort to let go of physical and emotional clutter, no matter how small, will yield rewards. As if by its own accord, you may find your practice starts to deepen, roadblocks fall away, old injuries disappear, and wonderful new things start to appear in your life.

But don't take my word for it. This spring (or whenever you read this), try it for yourself.

Stay Cool: Beat the Summer Heat

"Heat cannot be separated from fire, or beauty from The Eternal."
—Dante Alighieri

Before yoga, I used to struggle in the summer and would joke that I had reverse seasonal affective disorder (SAD). When I got overheated I'd become irritable, anxious, and unmotivated.

But it's no joke. According to the National Alliance on Mental Illness, just under ten percent of people in the U.S. with SAD suffer from symptoms of summer depression, which can include loss of appetite, trouble sleeping, weight loss, and anxiety.

My summer blues peaked during Chicago's infamous heat wave in July of 1995. I'd finally scraped together enough money to buy my first air conditioner and had installed it in the bedroom window of my stifling third-floor Wrigleyville apartment. That night I went to a nearby party, where we socialized outside until the neighborhood suddenly went pitch black. I rode my bike home in the eerie humid darkness and was dismayed to see that my block was also out of power, my new air conditioner rendered useless in the 100-plus degree heat. So I camped out on the floor—the coolest spot I could find—and cried myself to sleep. The power in Wrigleyville stayed off for three days, affecting 41,000 customers. The heat wave lasted five days and contributed to the deaths of 750 Chicagoans.

Two years later, I walked into my first yoga class—and began collecting the tools that have helped me handle the heat ever since. Some were picked up, while others come from my own experience. Perhaps they can help you, too.

Practice

Don't skip yoga! But try to avoid doing a lot of heat-building sun salutations or *vinyasas* (flowing poses) when it's extremely hot, and try a slower, more internal yoga practice with longer holds. Focus on wide-legged standing poses, side bends, and lying twists.

For a couple of summers, I attended the summer Guru Purnima program at a North Carolina ashram, where it was inevitably incredibly hot and humid in July. One of the program highlights was Sister Leslie's restorative yoga class, which always left me feeling cool and refreshed. Restorative poses are held for three to 10 minutes and are usually done with props such as bolsters and blankets. They can include supported child's pose, *salamba supta baddhakonasana* (supported supine bound angle), supported *janu sirsasana* (head-to-knee pose), and, of course, *savasana* (corpse pose)—the longer the better.

Whatever type of yoga you practice, don't neglect inversions. Poses such as shoulderstand and *viparita karani* (legs-up-the-wall pose) can be very cooling, especially if they are held for three minutes or longer. You can start out holding the pose as long as is comfortable, and then add several breaths (or 30 seconds) each time you practice.

If you feel too tired to practice, just do savasana. A savasana of twelve minutes or longer is a wonderfully detoxifying antidote to anxiety, depression, and fatigue and can make you feel like you've gotten a couple hours of sleep. (I like to practice it at home using Chandra Om's soothing 22-minute *Savasana* CD.)

To cool down quickly, do several rounds of *shitali pranayama* (cooling breathing). It was so hot when I taught at a local park one summer that we started class with this breathing practice and cooled down immediately (it also works for hot flashes). Sit in a comfortable position with the head, neck, and spine in a straight line. Roll the tongue into a tube and inhale through it. Then exhale through the nose. Repeat seven times (if you cannot form a tube, simply breath in through your teeth, and exhale through the nose).

Do deep, full diaphragmatic (belly) breathing throughout the day, especially if the heat causes you to feel anxious, lethargic, or mentally sluggish.

Diet

Lightening your diet can improve your energy level. Increase your intake of fruit, raw vegetables, and fresh juices, and reduce warming foods such as meat, poultry, fish, eggs, brown rice, beets, and sweet potatoes. Cooling fruits and vegetables include melon, banana, coconut, cucumber, avocado, broccoli, cauliflower, lettuce, and sprouts. (For maximum nutrient absorption, fruit and fruit juices should be consumed alone and on an empty stomach, and juice should be freshly squeezed.) If you have trouble breathing when the air quality is poor, reduce your intake of meat, wheat, and dairy.

Try adding cilantro, lime juice, and shredded coconut to cool down warm foods such as soups and kitchari (a stew made of moong dal and basmati rice; see "Kitcheri, Yoga's Wonder Food"), and cook them in coconut oil. Other cooling seasonings include mint, saffron, fennel, and dill. To cool down quickly, drink a glass of raw coconut water (ideally before 3:00 p.m. at room temperature).

Generally, heavy spices should be avoided, as they create more heat. But if your brain slows down when it's hot and humid, adding cayenne pepper to food can improve mental sharpness.

For a light, satisfying, high-protein breakfast, try Dharma's Breakfast Blend: eight to 12 ounces of coconut water blended with a handful of sprouted, peeled almonds; a handful of pineapple chunks; and half a banana. (To sprout the almonds, soak raw almonds in water overnight, then drain and place in a bowl covered with a damp towel for twelve hours. Peel before storing them in water, then refrigerate. Change the water every two days.)

Lifestyle

Stick to a schedule. Overcome the temptation to stay out late. Instead, go to bed and get up at the same time each day, and eat at regular times. If you suffer from insomnia, avoid heavy food after 6:00 p.m.

Try to make peace with the heat. Rose and sandalwood are naturally cooling scents. They can be found in essential oils, soaps, and incense. From time to time, take a stroll outside away from air conditioning. The early morning is the best time to do this. When you're inside, wear a shawl or light sweater in air-conditioned settings (to avoid shocking the body).

If the heat makes you tired, try speaking less (even to your pets). Also, observe how your pets and other animals react to intense heat. When it's very hot, they do less. So should humans. Learn to s-l-o-w down, and remember that you don't have to say yes to every invitation and obligation. When in doubt, say, "Let me think about it."

If your yoga clothes start to smell bad—even high-end, high-performance clothes can reek of mildew if you leave them to fester—try presoaking them in a solution of two cups of white vinegar and water (or in baking soda and water) before washing them. Or use an anti-odor detergent, such as 2Toms Stink Free Laundry Detergent or WIN High Performance Sport Detergent. Better yet, trade in the petroleum-based fabrics for natural, loose-fitting cotton.

Switch out the heavy shoes for sandals or flip-flops. (Back in the day, I'd wear combat boots year-round—even in summer. I looked cool, but didn't feel it. No wonder I was irritable!)

If all else fails, jump in the lake. Or a river. Or a pool—or at least through a sprinkler. It works every time.

Summer Tapas: Guru Purnima

*"Austerity involves seeking out discomfort
for the sake of personal growth."*
—Yogi Cameron

What are you putting off that would deepen your yoga practice?

Is it cleaning up your diet? Devoting ten minutes a day to meditation? Stopping bed-texting and spending time to reflecting upon the day's events? Working on a certain pose on a regular basis?

Rather than putting it off indefinitely, consider committing to a new level of practice for a four-month period, starting on Guru Purnima, a full moon day that occurs in July or August in the Hindu month of Ashad (a quick online search will reveal the current year's date).

Guru Purnima is a special day in which yogis commit to deepening their practice in order to honor their spiritual preceptor and all spiritual preceptors dating back to the sage Vyasa, who edited the *Vedas, Puranas, Srimad Bhagavatam,* and *Mahabharata.*

The guru is considered to be a living example of yoga, a saintly person who shares the practices that can bring the dedicated disciple face-to-face with God. On Guru Purnima, devotees may get up early and spend the day fasting, praying, and singing their guru's praises. Of course, the best way to honor the guru is to follow his or her teachings and achieve the goal of yoga: Self-realization (see "The Guru-Disciple Relationship").

Whether you have a guru or not, Guru Purnima gives yogis a wonderful opportunity to reaffirm their commitment to their spiritual practice, knowing that others around the world are doing the same thing. The collective consciousness is a powerful aid.

On this day, yogis make a commitment called a *sankalpa,* or a sacred vow. This vow is traditionally kept for a *chaturmas,* or four-month period.

A sankalpa made on Guru Purnima is not like a typical New Year's resolution, where one makes a vague, lofty plan that is followed for a few days and is then jettisoned as old habits reappear. Instead, it is a specific goal with a detailed plan on how to attain it. It is written down, signed, and then given to a spiritual preceptor or teacher.

This practice is part of the yogic observance of *tapas,* or purifying austerities. Tapas falls into three categories: austerity, worship, and charity, and can involve discipline of the body, speech, or mind. It can include practices to be taken up or habits to be given up.

Swami Sivananda said, "That which purifies the impure mind is tapas. That which regenerates the lower animal nature and generates divine nature is tapas. That which cleanses the mind and destroys lust, anger, greed etc., is tapas. That which destroys tamas (dullness) and rajas (impurity) and increases satva (purity) is tapas."

What you choose to do for Guru Purnima should be something that is reasonable given your particular circumstances. It should also be somewhat challenging. Usually, we have an idea floating around the back of our minds. If that is the case, write it down and visualize how it could be put into action. Remember, it should be appropriate for your particular stage of spiritual practice, and that yoga is, ultimately, about authentically wanting to clean up your act.

Once you figure out what your commitment will be, write it down, sign it, and put it into practice—not just for the guru or teacher, but also for your own spiritual unfoldment.

Because the real guru is right there, seated in your own heart, as your inmost Self.

Choosing and keeping your sankalpa

The more specific you are about your vow, the easier it will be to follow through. Include the steps you will take to accomplish it when you write it down. Sign it and give it to someone you believe in. (If you skip this last part, you are likely to fail.) Then, keep quiet about it and do the work.

If you do not have any ideas, here are a few places to start:

Give up a bad habit that is not serving you, such as bed-texting, having a glass of wine before bed, eating junk food, gossiping, or spending time with people who bring out the worst in you.

Spend five minutes a day reading the *Yoga Sutras* or other scripture.

Keep a daily spiritual diary, and write down your practices and how well you kept (or didn't keep) *yama*, yoga's ethical foundation. For more ideas, see "Keeping a Spiritual Diary" or read Swami Radha's 1996 book, *Time to Be Holy*.

Repeat a certain number of rounds of *mantra* each day, using a *mala* (a 108-bead rosary used for meditation). "A rosary is a whip to goad the mind towards God," said Swami Sivananda in his book *Japa Yoga*.

Develop a home practice. Resolve to do 20 minutes of *asana* (poses), 12 rounds of *pranayama*, and/or 10 minutes of meditation each day. Or promise yourself that you'll go to class a certain number of times each week.

Give up eating meat. If this seems too drastic, consider cutting it out of your diet once or twice a week (for more info, visit meatfreemondays.com or vrg.org).

If you are not yet ready to deepen your yoga practice, perhaps there is something in your life that needs to be resolved first. Consider diving into that project you've been avoiding, such as putting your finances or house in order, or clearing out a practice space in a bedroom or corner of the living room.

Consider volunteering once a week or a couple of times a month; this selfless service, or *Karma* yoga, should be performed without attachment to results. For example, resist the urge to brag about it or put it on your résumé. For ideas, visit volunteermatch. org or read Ram Dass's 1985 book, *How Can I Help?*

Take a weekly Internet and smartphone break, or practice silence once a week. Or vow to eat a meal in silence with no TV, no talking, no texting, and no reading once a day or once a week.

Give away one object you no longer use each day or week. Give the items to charity, or post them on freecycle.org.

If you have a tendency to run behind schedule (i.e., you are always late), vow to arrive ten minutes early to each of your appointments.

Put the *Yoga Sutras* into practice. Read Yogi Cameron's book *The One Plan: A Week-by-Week Guide to Restoring Your Natural Health and Happiness.* And do the exercises.

Warming Up to Fall Weather

"Autumn is a second spring when every leaf is a flower."
—Albert Camus

A friend who lives in San Francisco once told me that she feels cold much of the time and wears a down jacket to ward off the morning chill, even in the summer.

"What do you eat?" I asked.

Turns out the primary foods in her diet are lentil soup and salads. I suggested that she try swapping lightly steamed vegetables for the salads and start adding brown rice to her lentils (brown rice is warming) and then notice if it made a difference. Because what you eat affects how you feel.

In the northern climates, the cold season's dry wind and dipping temperatures can lead to a *vata* imbalance, or too much air or wind in the body. According to yoga's sister science, *ayurveda*, an overabundance of vata can manifest as dry skin; difficulty keeping warm; joint pain; anxiety and restlessness; weight loss; poor circulation; insomnia; rigid thinking; fearfulness; dizziness; or gas, flatulence, constipation, and other digestive problems.

In addition, many people suffer from seasonal affective disorder (SAD) during the dark months. SAD symptoms include low energy, depression, mood swings, oversleeping, overeating (especially a craving for high-carb foods), weight gain, and an overall feeling of hopelessness.

I tend towards the vata category; as soon as autumn hits, I get chilled easily, my skin becomes dry, my digestion slows down, my body becomes stiff, and my mind becomes anxious. That's when I know it's time to switch to my cold-weather diet and lifestyle. I learned how to do this after ending up in the emergency room with blocked digestion several years ago; afterward I called my mentor, Chandra Om, founder of the Shanti Niketan Ashram and author of *The Divine Art of Nature Cure.* She made some suggestions that immediately restored me to health. Some of what follows was learned from her and from my guru, Sri Dharma Mittra; I've relied on my own experience and other sources as well.

Yoga is experiential, so don't take my word for any of these things. Try one or two for yourself, and see if they work. If they do, hang on to them. If not, let them go.

Diet

When cold weather hits, it can feel like something's stuck—and not just the bowels. That's when it's time to reignite the digestive fire. For centuries, yogis have done this—and cleaned the stomach—by drinking a cup of warm water with the juice of half a lemon first thing in the morning. In the cold months, a few sprinkles of cayenne pepper may be added to help heat things up. If you're feeling congested, add ginger and turmeric. The concoction may be sweetened with maple syrup, honey, agave nectar, or whatever is handy.

It's important to eat at the same time each day, which is especially important for a vata imbalance. Avoid eating heavy food after 6:00 p.m. (eating heavy food late at night can interrupt sleep and make the body feel stiff and heavy in the morning). If your digestion is slow, avoid eating too much dairy, meat, wheat, or leftover/processed food. Increase water intake and certain live foods such as pineapple, plums, spinach, and oranges to alleviate constipation, but avoid salads, which cool the digestive fire; substitute lightly steamed vegetables. (For more, read "The C Word: Help for Constipation").

You can also combat excessive vata energy with fresh (not leftover), moist, warming, grounding foods such as soup, stews made with root vegetables, and kitchari, a digestion-friendly stew made of moong dal and rice (see "Kitchari, Yoga's Wonder Food"). Just don't skimp on the oil, which lubricates your digestive system.

Try baked sweet potatoes slathered with ghee or olive oil, oatmeal with plump raisins that have been soaked in water for 20 minutes, or butternut squash soup. Cooking at home, rather than going out, will result in healthier meals. It's also a great way to warm up and reduce stress.

Use plenty of ghee or organic olive oil and warming spices such as cardamom, cumin, ginger, cinnamon, salt, cloves, mustard seed, basil, oregano, sage, tarragon, thyme, and black pepper. Avoid sprouts, salads, most beans, tofu, cabbage, popcorn, toast, crackers, chips, and any other cold or gas-producing foods. Limit coffee intake as well as barley, corn, millet, and rye.

If you have trouble sleeping, reduce your caffeine intake, and avoid it altogether after 3:00 p.m. Instead, try warming ginger tea.

Lifestyle

To balance symptoms of vata, go to bed and get up at the same time each day, and build some downtime into your schedule. Add more bright and warming colors to your wardrobe and home. After attending my Beat the Winter Blues workshop, a student started using brightly colored plates in the winter and claimed that it immediately cheered her up. The most warming colors are red, orange, yellow, and pink. But any bright color will cheer you up (colors such as black, gray, and navy blue may be stylish, but they are not warming).

Wear warm clothes at home and outside. If you have trouble sleeping, try wearing a hat and socks (I do).

If your house is drafty, invest in a safe space heater. I take mine with me from room to room when the temperature dips below zero, and unplug it when I leave.

Spend time outside whenever you can, even if it's just a walk to mail a letter. Nature is the great healer, and the sun's natural light— even on cloudy days—will give you a dose of vitamin D and help regulate your internal timeclock. Sit in the sun whenever possible (but protect your skin if you're staying out for a long time).

If you can't go outside, visit a conservatory or botanic garden (or even a florist with a greenhouse). My friend and I did this during a particularly grueling winter, and the beautiful flowers and greenery immediately warmed us up, opened up our sinuses, and made us feel human again.

During the flu season, keep in mind that 99 percent of all illness is related to stress. Yoga of course is a wonderful de-stressor.

But it's also important to weave regular periods of relaxation or "doing nothing" into our schedules. I call it "enforced periods of relaxation." It can be as simple as sleeping in once in a while, spending time in nature, or taking a longer *savasana* (final resting pose; see below).

To soothe the skin and joints and induce sleep, take a hot bath before bed. Pour in a few teaspoons of sesame oil (made from un-toasted sesame seeds) and Epsom salt.

Practice

Don't neglect asana practice! If you're depressed or suffering from SAD, make sure you attend class; do not stay home and practice. Being with other people will remind you that you're not alone. Helpful poses for SAD include twists and backbends. In general, a more active practice (such as Ashtanga or Vinyasa) is recommended for those experiencing lethargy or depression.

If your digestion has stalled, be sure to include plenty of slow meditative twists, forward bends, deep squats, and belly-down backbends such as cobra, *salabasana* (locust), and *dhanurasana* (bow) to help get things moving. Traditional poses to aid digestion such as the half wind-relieving pose (with the thigh pressed into the belly) can also help. Do not skip savasana, and stay there for at least seven minutes.

Those who know *bhastrika,* or bellows breath, and positive breathing should include those as well. Deep breathing will also help (see "Change Your Breathing, Change Your Life"). Better yet, go to class so your teacher can show you these things in person.

That said, practice the first ethical rule of yoga—*ahimsa,* or nonharming—and stay away from class when you're sick and can infect others. In general, people are contagious one day before and two to three days after common cold symptoms appear, and for flu, it's one day before to a week after symptom onset, so consider doing a short, easy home practice and take rest if you're feeling run down. And don't forget: If you can't breathe, it will be extremely difficult to practice yoga.

Weathering Winter Gracefully

"The sun did not shine. It was too wet to play.
So we sat in the house. All that cold, cold, wet day."
—Dr. Seuss, *The Cat in the Hat*

Many of us have difficulty transitioning to the cold weather, especially as we age. But yoga and ayurveda have time-tested methods that can make things go more smoothly during the darkest, coldest days of the year.

Winter is the time to quiet down, do less, and "be" more—to go within. In other words, to make practice a priority. If you've been putting off starting a meditation practice, now is the time to take it up, when the stillness of winter is working in your favor.

Regular yoga practice—including poses, *pranayama* (breathing), concentration/meditation, and relaxation—strengthens the immune system and gives us a solid foundation to face the long winter. If time is limited, sun salutations are the ideal way to warm up and loosen the body in the morning. Follow them up with some of the main poses, such as cobra/backbend, *paschimottanasana* (seated forward bend), headstand, shoulderstand, spinal twist, and a *savasana* (final rest) that is at least seven minutes long.

Make sure you breathe deeply when you practice, because the breath contains *prana*, the essential life force. Diaphragmatic breathing improves digestion, brain function, and posture; increases energy; and reduces stress. Make sure the inhale is as long as the exhale, and that the belly is moving. Adding *ujjayi*, or victorious breath, by making a gentle snoring or hissing sound in the back of the throat creates heat, draws the mind's attention to the breath, and automatically has a calming effect.

Motivation can go out the window in winter. To make sure you stick to your practice, it is good to make a *sankalpa*. A sankalpa is not a resolution; it is a solemn vow. To make a sankalpa, write down your intention at the top of a piece of paper and below write exactly how you will do it (for example, "Meditate regularly for ten minutes, five days a week, for the rest of winter"). Sign your sankalpa and give it to someone you trust—or burn it. Keep a copy for yourself, and look at it from time to time to see how you're doing. A sankalpa is like a contract with yourself, and it is important to stick to it.

The body craves a steady supply of fresh, warm, healthy food in winter. Avoid foods that are processed, canned, frozen, reheated, or packaged, as they can make you tired and tax the immune system. Also stay away from cold drinks. Try drinking herbal tea or hot water with lemon rather than caffeinated beverages, which can increase anxiety, dehydrate the body, and make it difficult to sleep.

Warm, sweet, moist, nourishing foods keep the body warm and grounded. These can include steamed, baked, or roasted sweet potatoes slathered with healthy oil and soups made with seasonal items such as butternut squash. For breakfast, try a bowl of organic oats cooked with fennel and cardamom and served with raisins that have been soaked in water for 20 minutes (this makes them plump and moist). Buckwheat and quinoa are also wonderfully warming, energy-producing breakfast foods, especially when cooked with nuts. Kitchari, a combination of moong dal and rice, has been eaten by yogis for centuries and is very warming and nourishing when made with brown basmati rice. It is also easy to digest (see "Kitchari, Yoga's Wonder Food").

Oil is one of the best antidotes to dry, cold weather. If you suffer from dry skin, try pouring a few teaspoons of uncooked sesame oil into your bath at night. If the body is stiff, add a cup of Epsom salt. After the bath, rub a few drops of sesame oil into the nostrils and ears to relieve dryness.

Make sure you also include plenty of oil in your diet to lubricate the joints, aid digestion, and keep the bowels working properly. Olive oil is good for most body types. For stiffness, my guru, Sri Dharma Mittra, recommends consuming two tablespoons of raw flaxseed oil or hemp nut oil or a 3-6-9 blend of flaxseed, sesame, and sunflower seed oils before breakfast.

If you get depressed in winter, try adding some bright, warming colors to your wardrobe, such as red, pink, orange, or yellow. Put up a string of holiday lights—and leave it up until winter ends. Spend a few minutes of each day outside while the sun is out (whether you can see it or not). If possible, spend time in nature once or twice a week. Just make sure you're wearing a hat, a warm jacket, and plenty of layers.

If you get chronically tired during the dark months, learn to stop saying yes to every invitation and build more quiet time into your schedule. Go to bed a little earlier than usual so that you get enough rest.

Most important, keep practicing yoga. Recent studies have shown that regular yoga practice can greatly reduce symptoms of clinical depression. "The more the participants attended yoga classes, the lower their depressive symptoms at the end of the study," said Dr. Maren Nyer, who conducted a 2017 pilot study at Massachusetts General Hospital. She also found that it improved the participants' sense of optimism.

Part Three: Yoga Lifestyle

Developing a Home Practice

"The secret to success in yoga is constant practice."
—Sri Dharma Mittra

Sometimes, we don't have time, energy, or money to go to a yoga class.

Sometimes, we just need to get on the mat at home and figure things out for ourselves.

But it can be difficult to tune out all of the distractions at home; there are dishes to wash, bills to pay, e-mails to check.

The other roadblock is figuring out exactly *what* to practice. It's easy if you have a sequence to follow, such as the Ashtanga Vinyasa yoga sequence or the series of poses presented in the back of BKS Iyengar's *Light on Yoga*. Sometimes, though, it's nice to just get on the mat and see what happens.

What I'm certain of is this: When I practice, the arrows that life shoots at me are deflected. When I don't practice, each one hits its target.

Here are some other tips that may help you:

1. Set up a special place to practice

Swami Sivananda said, "Have a separate meditation room under lock and key. If this is not possible, then a corner of the room should be set apart with a small cloth screen or curtain drawn across. Keep the room spotlessly clean." The *Hatha Yoga Pradipika* says, "The Yogi should practice Hatha Yoga in a small room, situated in a solitary place, being 4 cubits square, and free from stones, fire, water, disturbances of all kinds, and in a country where justice is properly administered, where good people live, and food can be obtained easily and plentifully."

Putting aside the question of justice, I recommend setting up an altar and placing what you like on it. What inspires you? Patanjali? Jesus? Your grandmother? Do you like candles? Incense? It's ideal if you face east when you practice; north is a good second choice. But don't get bogged down in the details. My practice space is in the corner of the living room, with a small altar in a bookcase featuring pictures of my guru and other influential teachers. I keep my yoga mat out where I can see it; that way, it's like an open invitation to sit and/or do *asana* (yoga postures/poses). This has virtually eliminated my tendency toward procrastination. That said, you can practice anywhere there's space––even if it requires moving some furniture.

2. Do what you can with the time that you have

Make time to practice. And remember, it's better to practice a little bit every day than once a week for three hours. In other words, every asana practice need not be 90 minutes long. Sometimes, we only have 15 minutes. This is enough time for a brief sit, or sun salutations, or *savasana* (corpse pose). It's better to do something than nothing. If you can sit in meditation for five minutes each day, that's wonderful. If you can do it at the same time each day, even better. Just make sure you practice nonattachment, and take a day off from asana practice at least once a week.

Once you get on the mat, don't get off until you're done—no matter what. As Sri Dharma Mittra says, "You have to make some effort."

Students often ask what time of day they should practice. The short answer is: whenever you can, as long as the bowels and stomach are empty. If the only time you can practice is noon, then that's when you should practice. My guru, Sri Dharma Mittra, says that the best time to practice asana is 4:00 p.m., when the body is warm. But most people are at work at that time.

Traditionally, the optimum time for meditation is at Brahma-muhurta (about an hour and a half before sunrise—roughly 4:00 to 6:00 a.m.), and again at midday and sunset; in India, the Ashtanga asana practice is done early in the morning when the air is clean and cool. But that might not be a most comfortable or convenient time for you. As TKV Desikachar relates in his book *Health, Healing, and Beyond: Yoga and the Living Tradition of Krishnamacharya,* his father, Tirumalai Krishnamacharya, was devoted to reconciling the received knowledge with modernity. "One practices in India early in the morning because only then is it cool enough for comfort. This would be entirely inappropriate in Switzerland in winter—midday would then be best."

3. Don't procrastinate
Turn off the phone. Step away from the computer. And trick yourself if you must.

Checking e-mails and washing the dishes can wait; as the first Yoga Sutra says, "Now begins the practice of yoga"—not 20 minutes from now or next week. As Swami Sivananda used to say, "D.I.N."(Do it now!). Procrastination leads to thinking, which is the enemy of yoga, where the goal is to quiet the mind.

I'm a veteran procrastinator and used to have to trick myself into home practice. Even though I'd be wearing my pajamas or street clothes, I'd say to myself, "I'll just move this chair out of the way and do one sun salutation right here on the bare floor and see how it feels." Without fail, one sun salutation turned into two and then three and more, and soon, I'd be pulling out the mat and doing an entire 90-minute practice. So tell the mind you're only going to do one. And see what happens.

4. Have a plan/goal in mind
Feeling depressed and low on energy? Maybe it's a good day to work on sun salutations, backbends, and spinal twists. Anxious? Forward bends and long, supported poses may help. If the body is really depleted, *yoga nidra* could be just the thing to restore your energy. If you have a half hour, perhaps several rounds of sun salutations and a sitting practice would be best.

Find a sequence that you like, or create one yourself. Research websites and books, and figure out a plan. TKV Desikachar's excellent 1999 book, *The Heart of Yoga: Developing a Personal Practice,* explains exactly how to construct a practice. You could also loosely follow the Asthanga model, starting with warm-ups, followed by standing poses, seated poses, backbends, and inversions. Or the classical Hatha yoga method: sun salutations, headstand, shoulderstand and plow, backbend, forward bend, spinal twist, and savasana.

Another option is to work towards a nemesis pose, doing warm-ups and easier variations before finally attempting the full pose; I've done this with several seemingly impossible poses, and eventually mastered them (others, however, have mastered me).

Or try to repeat what you can remember from the last time you took a class. Another option is to simply get on the mat and see what happens. Just don't forget *savasana* (final rest); it's perhaps the most important posture, and skipping it can unsettle the mind. Try to stay in it for at least seven minutes.

5. Include at least one pose you don't like or that's difficult for you

Breathe slowly while you're in your nemesis pose. Then, see if you can do it one or two more times. Go a little deeper each time, as long as your breathing is smooth and even. As Sri Dharma Mittra says, "The way to develop strong willpower is to do the things you find distasteful." Just make sure you practice first precept of yoga, *ahimsa*—that is, don't hurt yourself.

6. Experiment!

Try some things you learned in class. Find out what works and what doesn't work. Since no one's looking, why not try lotus with your left foot first (as long as it doesn't hurt your knees)? Play with sequences. Or practice with a friend. My friend Michael and I did this once; he called out a pose, and we went into it. Then it was my turn to call out a pose. We did this for two hours. It ended up being a playful, eclectic practice that took me way, way outside of my self-practice comfort zone.

My body is rather lopsided, and I find it helpful to do my "tight" side twice in a pose, or to hold the tight side twice as long as the "open" side. This is something one rarely gets to do in a class with other people, and it can help even out imbalances in the body.

7. Develop a sitting practice

Theoretically, we do all these yoga poses so that the body is comfortable sitting still. It can take as little as five minutes a day to develop a sitting practice (and it works even better if it takes place after an asana practice). Simply turn off all electronic devices and find a comfortable, steady seat. Then you can focus on *trikuti* (the space between the eyebrows, behind the forehead). Or watch the breath (which is different from controlling the breath). Or do any concentration/meditation practice that you like (in this case, it's usually best to avoid the practices you don't like). And stick with it.

It's not necessary to do lotus or even sit on the floor; you may use a chair if that's where you're most comfortable. As long as your back is straight and the nape of the neck is in line with the spine, it doesn't matter where you sit.

If you have a *pranayama* (breathing) practice, do it before your concentration/meditation practice. Start the whole thing with one or three Oms (actually, "Oming" over and over is a practice in itself and can make you feel really, really good); if you have the time, add one minute per week to your sitting practice. Soon, you'll be sitting for half an hour.

An effective sequence is: Om or mantra, followed by asana, savasana, pranayama, and concentration/meditation.

8. Do it because it has to be done

Try not to be attached to the outcome of your practice. Offer it up to God or someone you love or something that's dear to your heart. You'll still receive all the benefits. As the *Bhagavad-Gita* says, "Remaining steadfast in yoga, O Dhananjaya, perform actions, abandoning attachment, remaining the same to success and failure alike. This evenness of mind is called yoga."

If this doesn't resonate with you, consider how wretched the body and mind feel when you skip practice!

9. Take a class from time to time

It's easy to pick up bad habits when you practice at home all the time. You get sloppy, become stagnant, lose all sense of alignment, or hold the poses you don't like for just a few breaths (or, worse, avoid them altogether). A good teacher will correct your mistakes, challenge you, inspire you, and keep you honest.

Keeping a Spiritual Diary

*"You have to light your own lamp. No one will give you salvation.
I am talking of enlightenment. All individuals have the
responsibility to enlighten themselves. Do not think you
cannot do it. You have that spark. You are fully equipped.
You simply need to discipline yourself. Discipline is not a prison.
It simply means practice."*
—Swami Rama

Many years ago I decided I wanted to be a journalist but didn't know how to go about doing it. I felt overwhelmed because it seemed like such a monumental undertaking. I was stuck until someone close to me suggested I work on my new career for ten minutes a day, every day. "I can do that," I thought. And I did do it—eventually earning a Master's degree in journalism and enjoying a successful career in Chicago media.

Decades later, I decided I wanted to master *hanumanasana*, the splits. I worked on it a little bit every day, and sure enough, soon I was doing the splits.

The same holds true for any yoga practice that one wishes to master—especially the higher practices of concentration and meditation—particularly if one is not attached to the outcome.

In the *Yoga Sutras*, Patanjali says "Practice (abhyasa) means choosing, applying the effort, and doing those actions that bring a tranquil state," and "When that practice is done for a long time, without a break, and with sincere devotion, then the practice becomes a firmly rooted, stable and solid foundation." (Sutras 1.13 and 1.14)

This flies in the face of today's cultural norms of instant gratification, reduced attention span, and general slovenliness. So many students come to class and want to see immediate results, and get turned off when they don't happen. Or they practice sporadically, or dabble in many different practices. But it is the consistent, day-in, day-out practice that yields the results.

And the three greatest obstacles to practice, according to yoga master Sri Tirumalai Krishnamacharya, are laziness, sleep, and disease.

My first teacher, Suddha Weixler, used to say that it is better to practice for a short time every day rather than once a week for a long period of time. And most spiritual teachers say it is best to stick to one tradition and do the same practice at the same time each day.

In other words, consistency is the key to success. As my guru, Sri Dharma Mittra, said in a 2014 *Yoganonymous* interview, "Do your meditation consistently as a way to turn the attention inward and away from the outer sense objects....

"I remember once I stopped doing everything unhealthy for three years. I had no contact with my family, I ate no cooked food, no candy, I didn't watch any movies and I went to the yoga class every day. After three years, I suddenly couldn't hold to that any longer. I went to 42nd Street where the movie theaters were with my pockets stuffed full of Reese's Peanut Butter Cups and Almond Joy bars. Almond Joy was my favorite! I went to the movies all day long.

"When you try to renounce too much all at once, that's what happens. You climb, and then you fall down hard. It's better to go slow, but to make steady progress."

As Sri Dharma notes, it can be difficult to maintain discipline and consistency over the long haul. But it is also essential, which is why keeping a spiritual diary can be so helpful.

"The spiritual diary is a whip for goading the mind towards righteousness and God," said Swami Sivananda. "If you regularly maintain this diary you will get solace, peace of mind and make quick progress in the spiritual path."

A spiritual diary can be a simple notebook or a Word document on your computer or a note on your phone—whatever is easiest for you. Make sure you record the date (including the year) at the top of each entry.

Then, note the practices you have done (or neglected!) each day. Also take time to reflect upon and write about any violation of *yama* and *niyama*, yoga's ethical roots. (A helpful book for learning how to do this is Swami Radha's *Time to be Holy*.) Her guru, Swami Sivananda, said, "By keeping a spiritual diary you can then and there rectify your mistakes. You can do more sadhana [practice] and evolve quickly. There is no other best friend and faithful teacher or Guru than your diary. It will teach you the value of time."

Even if you haven't done any practice, or have acted in a way inconsistent with the precepts of yoga, make sure to write in your diary every day. Be truthful. If you see a pattern of undesirable behavior, examine it, contemplate its cause, and then root it out.

"It is important to reflect about daily events and see how you would do something differently from how you did it last week," writes Swami Radha in *Time to Be Holy*. "By putting daily events in your diary and reflecting on them, you ensure that you will continue to work. That continuation will ensure your growth. The daily entry in your diary is actually the story of your spiritual development. It reflects the effort that you put in and, accordingly, what you will get in return. If your effort is very lukewarm then nothing will happen. If you notice in your reflection that you have repeated some mistake, you may think, 'Oh, I know all about this,' and because you know, you may think you don't need to pay more attention to it. But, you see, when we know things and then act contrary to what we know, that is a sin. Sin is not the mistakes we make. Sin is knowing what we have to do and not doing it."

She continues, "Even if you have failed in conquering your shortcomings for the fifth time, the tenth time, the twentieth time, you won't know about your failures if you don't put them down in your diary and examine them in your daily reflection. Then keep reading over the past months in your dairy, and you will see a lot of things coming together."

Keep all of your old spiritual diaries. When you are feeling discouraged or are lacking in enthusiasm, look back at what you were doing six months ago, a year ago, two years ago. And you will see that you are making real progress. Conversely, you may find that you are repeating the same old mistakes.

Just don't put it off. Start today.

Swami Rama said, "Discipline should not be forced by teachers or by others. Patanjali says the whole foundation of samadhi is *anushasanam*. You have to understand the word 'anushasanam' in a practical way. Discipline means to regulate yourself on three levels: mind, action, and speech. Determine that from today you will begin to discipline yourself. It is a simple thing. Do not make big plans or too many rigid rules for yourself. Start with small things: 'I will wake up at four-thirty.' One simple rule. 'After that, I will go to finish my ablutions and do my exercise. Exactly at five-thirty I will sit down in meditation.' Discipline yourself. If you do not have the zeal, vigor, and determination to discipline yourself, you cannot follow the path. When you have decided something, you need determination to act according to your decision. If you lack determination, you will not be successful, even though you have decided. If you have decided that you will practice yoga, that decision must be supported by determination. 'Yes. I will practice it every day. The day I don't practice, I will not eat.' The next day you will say, 'I have to practice because I have to eat.'"

But don't beat yourself up if you fail. Simply start over again. "Most important, if you lose your self-control, don't get angry," said Sri Dharma Mittra. "Sometimes, according to your deeds from the past, cravings and desires will torment you like hell. Just do your best. If for some reason the result is not the way you like, you have to be content. 'I did my best, my Lord.'"

Do One Thing at a Time

"For him who has conquered the mind, the mind is the best of friends; but for one who has failed to do so, his very mind will be the greatest enemy. For one who has conquered the mind, the Supersoul is already reached, for he has attained tranquility. To such a man happiness and distress, heat and cold, honor and dishonor are all the same."
—The *Bhagavad-Gita*

The second Yoga Sutra states "yogash chitta vritti nirodhah"; yoga is the settling of the mind into silence. The goal of Patanjali's Raja yoga is to quiet the mind so that the spark of the divine in each of us—the source of bliss and peace that is our true nature—can shine forth.

But before the mind can become quiet, it must learn to concentrate on a single object for a long period of time.

As Swami Sivananda says in his commentary on Yoga Sutra IV-20, the mind can jump from thought to thought with lightning speed, but it can only hold a single thought at a time.

"A spark of light presents the appearance of a continuous circle of light if it is made to rotate rapidly," he writes in *Raja Yoga*. "Even so, the mind, though it can attend to one thing at time, either hearing, seeing or smelling, though it can admit one kind of sensation at a time, we are led to believe that it does several actions at a time, because, it moves from one object to another with tremendous velocity, so rapidly, that its successive attention and perception appear as a simultaneous activity."

Think about it; the mind can hold only one thought at a time.

Yet we live in an increasingly fast-paced, multi-tasking society that operates at breakneck speed.

But when we multi-task, we are actually training the mind to do the opposite of yoga: to jump even more quickly from thought to thought. This reduces concentration and makes meditation more difficult or even impossible. It also makes our work difficult—we can actually become *less* productive (and make more mistakes) when we multi-task.

Worse, it further unsettles the mind, making it even more agitated and more difficult for us to experience the inner peace that is always there, waiting for us to notice.

In other words, multi-tasking can make us miserable. The mind can become our tormentor as it craves more and more stimulation, jumping from object to object, never happy with what it is experiencing in any given moment.

Fortunately, the mind can be trained.

We can retrain the mind to slow down and concentrate by doing one thing at a time. You can start with your next meal. Sit down at the table (not the couch) and eat it in silence, without reading, texting, talking, watching TV, or even daydreaming. You may find that the mind rebels, becoming incredibly bored and then begging for stimulation. But stick with it. Don't give in. Notice the flavor and texture of your food as you chew it. Give thanks to those who made it possible for you to eat it (the farmers, the grocers, those who transported it to you, etc.). And then keep pulling your mind back to your food and the sensations of biting, chewing, and swallowing as they occur. Remember that there will be some agitation at first, but eventually the mind will become quiet and peaceful and absorbed in its task.

One of the *Bhagavad-Gita*'s definitions of *sattva* (peace, purity, and harmony) is "That which is like poison in the beginning becomes like nectar in the end." The practice of doing one thing at a time can initially make the mind more rebellious, but it will calm down and become quiet and obedient if you stick with it.

Doing one thing at a time can be practiced with any activity—washing the dishes (no talk radio!), walking the dog (leave the phone at home!), waiting for the bus (no texting!), driving (no radio!), going to sleep (TV and phone switched off!), and so on.

Don't take my word for it, try it! You may find that after some initial turbulence, which can be rather unpleasant, you are more and more in the moment. You may even experience that wonderful feeling of peace that comes after a good yoga class.

It's also likely that your work will become easier as the mind relearns how to focus on one thing at a time.

You may also find that the mind, now under control, becomes your best friend.

Time Is Not on Your Side

"You have two hours to watch a movie, but no time to meditate?"
—Sri Dharma Mittra

It seems like in modern life we never have enough time—to practice, to get our work done, to see our friends and family.

But in yoga, time has always been of the essence.

Be a yogi. Be on time.

I remember seeing the "Be a yogi. Be on time." aphorism on the schedule at New York's original Jivamukti school in 1999 and thinking, "Yes, one should be on time for class." It wasn't until years later that I realized that being chronically late (one of my old habits) is a violation of *asteya,* or nonstealing, the third *yama,* or ethical foundation, of yoga.

Being late steals time from the others who are waiting for you, since their time is wasted and can never be returned to them. If you understand the laws of *karma* and reincarnation, you know that being late hurts you more than it hurts others, since you will eventually have to pay the price.

Nor is it good for your *asana* (postures) practice. It increases adrenaline and makes the heart beat fast. This causes the mind to become *rajasic* (passionate) rather than *sattvic* (calm). Only a sattvic mind can achieve Self-realization, which yogis believe is the highest goal in life.

The excitement produced by being chronically late can fuel the ego, one of the greatest obstacles to Self-realization. Constant tardiness can be addictive, especially for those who suffer from boredom or *tamas* (inertia). It also can make the powerless feel powerful, holding others hostage as they wait for the late one, who then makes a dramatic entrance filled with meaningless apologies.

If you are chronically late (in my experience, it is the same few people who are always late to class), take a few minutes for *svadhyaya* (self-study) and explore what you get from it. Because there has to be a reason; otherwise, why keep doing it? Is it the power? The rush? The drama? The fact that you get to constantly beat yourself up for failing others? Are you addicted to procrastination? Something else? Or are you *really* that busy?

Then act on what you find. Try giving yourself 10 minutes of extra time to get where you're going the next time you have an appointment, and see what happens.

You may find that the extra time leads to less road rage, less anger (directed at both others and yourself), and less frustration with entities such as the subway or bus system. You may find that you're bored out of your skull (many of us expend a great deal of energy trying to escape boredom, which is an obstacle to meditation); by living with the boredom, you will be able to transcend it.

And you may find something extraordinary: a calm mind. A calm body with less stiffness in the shoulders and neck. An even, comfortable breathing rhythm. A calm digestive system that can easily assimilate the food you've consumed.

In other words, a yogi's body and mind.

Stop wasting time

Yogis believe that two of the greatest gifts, not to be taken lightly or squandered, are human life and time. How do you spend your time? Do you use it to figure out and pursue your *dharma* (life's purpose), or do you waste it by pursuing entertainment and other transient sense-pleasures?

"The purpose of life is dharma," veteran teacher Aadil Palkhivala said at the 2011 Midwest *Yoga Journal* conference in Lake Geneva, Wisconsin. "Entertainment is a distraction from dharma."

How much time do you spend on entertainment? You know, looking up old friends on Facebook? Finding the perfect pair of shoes? Watching TV? Staring at your iPhone? Other forms of procrastination (like cleaning house when you should be working on a deadline)? How much time do you spend beating yourself up for wasting time? Or worse, complaining that you don't have enough time to do your yoga practice?

Have you ever calculated how much time you waste? Try setting a stopwatch the next time you're on the Internet or phone, and see where the time goes. And notice how wasting your time makes you feel. Then, calculate how much time you spend pursuing your dharma.

There's no way to know how much time we each have left. But at least we can control what we do in this very moment.

D.I.N.!

Many were surprised to learn at my 30th high school reunion that 10 percent of our class had already passed away. "One in ten!" people kept exclaiming. A candle was lit for each deceased classmate in front of his or her senior picture. It was impossible not to be moved. It also made for some unexpected introspection.

Many asked themselves: What do I want to accomplish before I die? What am I waiting for? How much time do I have left? What am I going to do with it?

Yogis believe each person is allotted a certain number of breaths at birth, according to their deeds from the past. Once they use up these breaths, it's time to leave this body. That's one of the reasons the science of yoga places such great importance on slow, measured breathing—so that there is time to accomplish your dharma, what you came here to do.

How to figure out your dharma? Turn off the TV, phone, and computer, and spend some time alone or in nature. Quiet the mind using such yogic techniques as *sattvic* diet (fresh, mild, vegetarian food), relaxation, control of the senses, concentration, and meditation. This will help you tune out the static and tune into your inner intuition, where the answer lies (if there's a question of whether the ego or intuition is guiding your actions, it is the ego). Or, analyze your past and present actions with a critical eye; what do you shy away from, and what do you gravitate towards? It's possible that your dharma lies with the latter.

If you are not ready to pursue your long-term goal, there may be work you need to do on yourself, such as going through therapy, straightening out your life, or putting your finances in order. But don't let it be an excuse not to pursue your long-term goals.

You can still start pursuing your dreams right now, even for just 10 minutes a day.

Be fearless and do not give in to doubts. If you're meant to do it, you cannot possibly fail, even if you stumble from time to time. Eventually, everything will fall into place to help you find your way. Just be sure not to violate *yamas* and *niyamas* (yogic observances), and to practice *Karma* yoga (selfless action, or offering up the fruits of your work) in the process.

If your dharma is to have children, find a suitable partner and build a nest. If it's to be a dentist, complete the prerequisites and start applying to school. If it's to have a yoga butt, get yours to class. Just don't be attached to the results.

If your dharma is the highest goal in life—to deepen your practice and pursue Self-realization—then turn off the TV, decline social invitations, and deepen your practice! If you don't know how, ask your teacher. (Teachers love such questions.) Make your goal your top priority, and make every effort to realize it. Then, pray for a guru with all of your heart.

And don't forget that no effort towards Self-realization ever goes to waste; if you don't reach the goal in this lifetime, yogis believe you will pick up where you left off next time around. (And, according to the laws of karma and reincarnation, if you leave this world with unfulfilled desires, you will be reborn in order to pursue them. That is why it is important to differentiate between your dharma and your desires; the former comes from your heart, and the latter from the ego. This is why yoga places such importance on desirelessness, egolessness, nonattachment, and selfless service.)

The *Bhagavad-Gita* says, "In this no effort is ever lost and no harm is ever done. Even very little of this dharma saves a man from the Great Fear."

Just don't let that be an excuse to waste time.

Make a resolution, write it down, sign it, and give it to someone who will hold you to it.

As my spiritual mother said at one of her New Year's retreats, "What you're thinking about doing tomorrow, do today. What you're thinking about doing today, do now."

Swami Sivananda put it even more succinctly several decades ago: "D.I.N." (Do it now)!

Facing Fear

"Once at Varanasi, as [Swami Vivekananda] was coming out of the temple of Mother Durga, he was surrounded by a large number of chattering monkeys. They seemed to be threatening him. Swamiji did not want them to catch hold of him, so he started to run away. But the monkeys chased him. An old sannyasin was there, watching those monkeys. He called out to Swamiji, 'Stop! Face the brutes!' Swamiji stopped. He turned round and faced the monkeys. At once, they ran away. "Many years later, Swamiji said: 'If you ever feel afraid of anything, always turn round and face it. Never think of running away.'"
—from *The Story of Vivekananda*

What is your greatest fear? Is it losing your job or your home? Not living up to your potential? Something else?

A related question is, what are you avoiding? Taking the next step on your career or spiritual path? Finishing a project you started long ago? Removing someone or something from your life who/that is holding you back? Moving to another state? It is likely that fear is the source of your worry and procrastination.

But what is the source of your fear?

In yoga, all fear can be traced back to the fifth *klesha*, or obstacle on the spiritual path. The fifth klesha is fear of death, or clinging to life. Even though we may not be consciously thinking about death, the fear is always there, lurking in the background. It manifests in very tangible ways, in the fears that we have. And if we ignore our fears or put off confronting them, they will only grow bigger and paralyze us. We also lose a lot of energy keeping them at bay. But when we confront our fears directly, they disappear, just like Swami Vivekananda's monkeys.

In Hatha yoga, we deal with our fears on the mat by mastering the poses that scare us; it could be *hanumanasana* (splits) or inversions such as headstand or balances like handstand. We approach these poses slowly and methodically, building up to them over a period of time and breathing slowly and fully throughout the process. And we learn to ignore the voice we heard over and over as children, telling us, "Don't do that—you'll break your neck!"

The yogi then employs these same skills off the mat, calmly and directly confronting their deepest fears. First, the fear must be named. Then the yogi uses the intellect to explore the fear and trace it back to its source. For example, a fear of losing one's job is a tangible expression of the fear of death. With no income, there is no money to buy food and one could, theoretically, starve. But a yogi continues with the self-analysis and realizes he or she has friends and family who will take care of them or help them find a new job. One traces the fear to its worst possible outcome, and then realizes that the scenario is not based in reality and puts it to rest.

Swami Sivananda said, "Fear is illusory; it cannot live. Courage is eternal, it will not die. Perils, calamities, dangers are the certain lot of every man who is a denizen of this world. Therefore, O Man! Fortify your mind with courage and patience. Fortitude, courage, presence of mind will sustain you through all dangers."

Worrying only increases fear; it is like praying for the thing we don't want, and in yoga we know how powerful the mind can be. Instead, we train the mind to stop worrying by replacing each fearful thought with the opposite one. For example, if you are afraid of losing your job, envision yourself working happily at your ideal career.

If a fear persists, there are tangible ways to confront it. Fear of growing old can be overcome by volunteering to help the elderly; fear of death by helping hospice patients or meditating in a cemetery; fear of poverty by helping the homeless; and so on. The key is to confront it, not avoid it.

In yoga, we use the breath to calm the mind. One of the simplest and most effective *pranayamas* (breathing practices) is learning to breathe slowly and deeply into the lowest lobe of the lungs. This practice, called calming breathing, is learned lying on the back with the hands on the belly, the tips of the middle fingers meeting just above the navel. Exhale completely. Then inhale into the belly area for a count of eight, allowing the middle fingers to separate. Hold the breath for a count of four. Then exhale for a count of eight, as the fingers move back together. Continue for five minutes or longer. Pranayama should be comfortable and graceful; if the 8-4-8 count is too intense, substitute 6-3-6.

Swami Sivananda suggests the following meditation for those who are paralyzed by fear: "Sit with closed eyes in the early morning. Meditate on courage, the opposite of fear, for half an hour. Think of the advantages of courage and the disadvantages of fear. Practice the virtue during the day. Feel that you actually possess courage to an enormous degree. Manifest it in your daily life. In some weeks or months fear will be replaced by courage. Repeat the formula 'Om courage' mentally, daily several times."

Irrational fears can be magnified by outside causes, such as the media; one solution is to avoid the news for a few weeks and notice if the fears diminish. Limiting time spent on the Internet and social media sites can also be helpful. Instead, spend that time in nature.

Diet also contributes to one's emotional state. My guru, Sri Dharma Mittra, says that animals experience fear and anger when they are slaughtered, and that when we eat meat we ingest those same emotions. If this applies to you, try going meat-free for a month, and see if there is a change in attitude.

Another helpful practice can be to look back at past personal crises and analyze how each situation was resolved (each *was* resolved, since you are here reading this). We soon realize that there is an unseen hand guiding us and helping us along our path, which has always helped us in the past and will continue to help us in the future. Is there any reason to think things won't turn out this time, too? We are never truly alone, bereft of assistance.

In every situation we have a choice: fear or faith. And those who study and understand yoga's laws of karma and reincarnation know that life unfolds the way it does for our own good. "Everything is moving perfectly," says Dharma Mittra.

Swami Vivekananda said something similar: "As long as we believe ourselves to be even the least bit different from God, fear

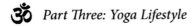

remains with us. But when we know ourselves to be the One, fear goes; of what can we be afraid?"

Cooperation vs. Competition

*"Regarding cooperation: it's good for you to try and lose yourself
a little—to move beyond the personal self and try and cooperate
with others. This really helps us understand that we are all one—
all part of the same great whole. The action of compassion is to
see yourself in others. If I see myself in you, how can I hurt you,
steal from you, or lie to you? Impossible! Learn to see yourself
in others and strive always to make every offering an act of
adoration to the Supreme Self or the forces behind everything.
Then we are all practicing yoga."*
—Sri Dharma Mittra, March 2017 issue of *Yoga Journal*

Yoga means union, or to yoke or join. To cooperate means to
"work jointly towards the same end," or to "assist someone or
comply with their requests," according to *The Oxford Living English
Dictionary.* Cooperation has its roots in love and compassion—or,
as Sri Dharma says, putting oneself in the place of others.

To compete means "to strive to gain or win something by de-
feating or establishing superiority over others," according to the
same source. Competition has its roots in the feeling of separateness,
which the *Yoga Sutras* of Patanjali cites as one of the main *kleshas,* or
causes of pain and suffering. Competing can actually reinforce and
strengthen this sense of isolation.

But practicing cooperation can sometimes feel like swimming upstream, especially when mainstream society often appears
to divide the world into "us" and "them" and reward unbridled
competition.

Indeed, I have struggled with these two poles for many years.

When I was in high school, I used to be the class cutup. One
day, one of my teachers got sick and tired of putting me out in

the hall to shut me up. After class, he explained to me that when I cracked jokes in class, he couldn't teach. He said he could no longer compete with me for the class's attention, and asked me to help him out by toning it down. Mortified, I immediately stopped making wisecracks (in *his* class, anyway).

Sri Dharma says, "Your worst enemy is your own self when you are not under control," but "When you are self-controlled, you like yourself."

Cooperation is something I continue to work on. But I have found that I am *always* happier when I let go of my habit of giving in to selfishness and try to cooperate with others. I inevitably suffer more when I compete (even though it may not initially feel that way, it *always* ends up that way). As Sri Dharma says, "Respect everything and divine love will flow through you very fast."

We can learn to cooperate in yoga class by respecting the body's limits on a given day, rather than competing with how our body was a decade or a week ago, or comparing our practice with that of the person next to us or someone on Instagram. My first teacher, Suddha Weixler, used to remind us regularly in class that "It's not a competition."

In yoga practice, when we compete, we end up either beating ourselves up mentally or forcing ourselves into a variation of a pose that causes pain—both of which are violations of yoga's golden rule, *ahimsa* (nonharming). Sri Dharma equates ahimsa to the *Bible*'s First Commandment, "Thou shalt not kill," explaining that it doesn't just apply to taking a life, but means, "Thou shalt not kill the comfort of others."

We can cooperate in class by moving together as a group rather than doing our own thing and distracting the rest of the people trying to follow along. One potential consequence of not cooperating is that new practitioners in class become confused and start following the person who's doing his or her own thing, which can result in injury. For some reason these lone wolves tend to put their mats in the front of the room, and, as a result, everyone else ends up having a diminished experience.

Sri Dharma often reminds us in class to "move together like a school of fish" in order to create a collective consciousness. "When you are doing things together, you are inside the collective mind, and share psychic knowledge with each other. That is how you become one."

When we move in and out of poses as he describes, the effect is incredibly powerful; everyone ends up benefiting more from their practice. (Sri Dharma also reminds us that the fish who goes off on her own is usually the one that is eaten by a bigger fish.)

Science is starting to back this up; studies show that cooperating with others can improve our self-esteem, sense of belonging, and overall health.

Cooperation results in more happiness and connection for everyone; competition magnifies the feeling that one is isolated and doing everything on one's own.

Cooperation benefits the group; competition benefits the individual.

The benefits of cooperation are infinite; the results of competition are limited.

I remember taking the noon master class with Sri Dharma at his old New York City studio in 1999 and being struck by the feeling of unity and love in the room. Instead of competition (for poses, for mat space, for attention, etc.), there was an overwhelming feeling of reverence and cooperation. I immediately felt accepted and supported by the rest of the group. Indeed, it felt like everyone else in the class was rooting for me and mentally helping me to do better. I found myself trying—and doing—poses I'd never thought possible. I also felt incredibly *good*—physically, mentally, and spiritually—during and after the class.

On the highest level, this type of cooperation in class means making every action an offering to the Supreme Self, the spark of the divine or pure consciousness that is common to everyone. In other words, seeing oneself in others. This type of cooperation is rooted in selflessness, or the yogic ideal of *isvara pranidhana* (surrender of the ego to the collective consciousness).

Sri Dharma often says, "If you see someone doing a nice pose, don't think, 'That is them.' Think, 'That is me.'" In other words, imagine that you are doing the pose through them. "If you see yourself everywhere, that is a sign of Self-realization," he says.

Whether you are able to do this or not, cooperating with your own body and the rest of the group makes for a better experience for everyone.

This type of cooperation can easily be carried off the mat and into daily life. It can be as simple as not disturbing your neighbors with loud music at night, or it can mean letting someone go ahead of you in line, not waving your fist at the sky when you're expecting good weather and it starts to rain, giving up your seat on the train for an elderly person, shoveling out an extra parking space the next time it snows, or even cutting vegetables along their natural growth lines (Maya Tiwari explains how to do the latter in her wonderful book *The Path of Practice: A Woman's Book of Ayurvedic Healing*). It can mean forgiving someone who chooses not to apologize or being the one who apologizes, even when you know you are in the right. The opportunities are only limited by our imagination and our ability to put ourselves in the place of others.

Nowadays, when I end a class, I share what Sri Dharma tells students: "Be receptive to the grace of God."

This grace, which is always there and is inexhaustible, flows more freely when we cooperate with each other. When we don't, it slows to a sad little trickle.

But don't take my word for it—try it and see for yourself.

Eight Great Movies About Yoga

I've seen many amazing movies about yoga over the years, but most don't even have "Yoga" in the title. Nonetheless, they provide a painless way to explore some of the core principles of yoga, or union with the divine.

Naked in Ashes

Despite the titillating title, Paula Fouce's riveting, beautifully shot 2005 documentary provides an intimate look at the lives of a handful of India's 13 million *sanyasis* (renunciates), who heal and provide spiritual instruction to seekers and own nothing—eschewing clothes even on pilgrimages through the snow. Today, these fierce-looking yogis are in danger of extinction. They tell their stories in their own words (nicely dubbed into English) and appear utterly at peace with enduring hardships, which helps them maintain focus on the divine. It's a wonderful reminder of the importance of *tapas* (self-discipline), *Karma* yoga (selfless service), *ishvara pranidhana* (surrender to God), and *vairagya* (nonattachment). Despite the film's poignancy (I was driven to tears more than once by the yogis' devotion), it also has many funny moments: I nearly fell off the couch when Shiv Raj Giri sweetly says that even after becoming a yogi, there is no peace. Indeed!

Groundhog Day

I learn something new each time I watch this 1993 comedy about an arrogant and cynical Pittsburgh weatherman (Bill Murray) who's trapped living the same day over and over again. Cited by some religious leaders as the most spiritual film of our time and shot in Woodstock, Illinois, it shows how egoism (*asmita*) makes us miserable and separates us from others. Murray's character is initially confused when he realizes his situation—then cunning, and then suicidal. After confiding in his producer and love interest, Rita (Andie MacDowell), he tries to improve himself—initially to impress her. It's only when his actions become truly selfless that his cynicism and ego disappear and he wins her heart, and finally stops reliving the same day. It's as if the film's message of selfless service was lifted directly from the *Bhagavad-Gita*: "To work alone you are entitled, never to its fruit."

Into Great Silence

This meditative 2005 film by Philip Gröning quietly follows six months in the lives of Carthusian monks at Chartreuse Monastery in the French Alps. These hermits spend most of their time alone in their cells, in study, silence, and contemplation. They get together for prayer services, but the only time they speak informally is during weekly walks in the stunningly beautiful countryside. The film, which utilizes natural light and sound and has little dialogue, has been called "one of the most mesmerizing and poetic chronicles of spirituality ever created," and shows the importance of *svadhayaha* (reading and reflecting upon sacred texts), *mauna* (silence), *mantra* (chanting), *dharana* (meditation), and *satsang* (keeping holy company). During and after watching this film, I felt as if I'd also spent time in the monastery: calm, centered, and incredibly *sattvic* (peaceful).

My Reincarnation

Tibetan Buddhist Master Choogyal Namkhai Norbu's Italian-born son, Yeshi, has been told since he was a child that he's the reincarnation of his father's uncle, a great master who was killed when China invaded Tibet. Yeshi has an uneasy relationship with his father, who fled Tibet in 1959 and wants his son to go there and meet the students who are waiting for him. Instead, the headstrong Yeshi focuses on career and a family and lives a worldly life. Filmmaker Jennifer Fox followed the pair for 20 years in this excellent 2010 documentary, which explores the conflict between *dharma* (duty), fate, and following one's own heart. In the end, Yeshi goes to Tibet, where he is warmly received, without telling his father. But then he returns home to become his father's student as well as a teacher in his own right.

Up!

This uplifting 3-D computer-animated film from 2009 follows a cranky widower named Carl (Ed Asner) who personifies the quality of *tamas* (inertia); he is negative, fearful, and set in his ways, and he clings to the past—living in the house that he and his wife built while the world around him has moved on (he also exemplifies two of yoga's greatest obstacles: *dwesha,* or aversion, and *raga,* or attachment). Carl meets a precocious boy and embarks on a grand adventure that proves one is never too old to follow a dream. But only when Carl lets go of his previously held notions and his most prized possession, his house, does a whole new world open up to him and life begin to take on new meaning. It's a fine example of the debilitating nature of tamas and the transformational power of vairagya.

Unmistaken Child

It can be difficult for the mind to accept yoga's laws of *karma* (spiritual principle of cause and effect) and reincarnation, but this exquisitely shot 2009 documentary helped remove many of my doubts. It follows a gentle 28-year old Nepalese monk named Tenzin Zopa on his four-year search for the reincarnation of his Tibetan guru, Geshe Lama Konchog, who died in 2001. Like any true master, Tenzin has no ego and believes he's not worthy of the task. But with his elders' urging, he scours rural Nepal looking for a young boy who is asked to pick out the lama's prayer beads from other beads, which the child is able to do. The quiet way the film deals with the guru-disciple relationship, which does not end with physical death but spans lifetimes, is especially disarming, particularly when Tenzin interacts with the child who was his master.

Vision: From the Life of Hildegard von Bingen

This extraordinary 2009 feature by Margarethe von Trotta focuses on the eleventh-century Benedictine abbess and mystic who went into the cloister at age eight (as a gift from her family) and took her vows at 16. When her spiritual mother and guru passes,

Hildegard is told to take over as prioress, but she won't do so until she is voted in by her sisters. Later she founds a couple of cloisters and writes books, musical compositions, and an early liturgical drama. She also travels to preach—unheard of for a woman at that time. Amidst the drama, the film touches on the guru-disciple relationship as well as the value of a life dedicated to work, spiritual study, healing, music, prayer, and meditation. It also explores what happens when one follows one's inner intuition in order to directly experience the divine. My favorite line in the movie occurs when Hildegard experiences doubt on the spiritual path: "The almighty has given you wings to fly. Fly over every obstacle."

Enlighten Up!

"Go f— yourself" is the last thing you'd expect to hear in this 2008 yoga documentary, but it's exactly what Norman Allen tells a skeptical Nick Rosen during the latter's six-month search for enlightenment (I think he was telling him to "Go within" to find the answers). Norman, who was the first American to study Ashtanga yoga with Pattabhi Jois, and lived with him for years, has some other choice words in this lively jaunt, which follows Nick from practicing with Dharma Mittra and Alan Finger and at Jivamukti Yoga School in New York City to practicing Yoga for Regular Guys in California (where the *dristi* [gaze] is not where you'd expect it to be) to studying with Pattabhi Jois, BKS Iyengar, and Swami Gurusharanananda in India. Each teacher has something to offer the skeptical Nick, but it's Norman, living in seclusion in Hawaii, who steals the show. When Nick asks him what the *asanas* (postures) have to do with the quest for enlightenment, he says, "Absolutely nothing."

Eight Great Yoga Memoirs

While many students of yoga have studied the *Yoga Sutras*, the *Bhagavad-Gita*, and the *Hatha Yoga Pradipika*, their key concepts can be difficult to grasp and even harder to put into practice. These teachings can come to life in the yoga memoir, especially those written by true yogis who admit to having fears and doubts along the way. I've found the following memoirs to be incredibly inspiring—and almost all emphasize the importance of the guru-disciple relationship.

Autobiography of a Yogi
by Paramahansa Yogananda

The first time I tried to read this 1946 classic, the mind decided it was BS and the hand flung it across the room. I read it again a few years later (for Sri Dharma Mittra's teacher training) and thought, "Yes, this is possible." The third time, I thought, "Of course!" This well-written memoir introduced yoga and meditation to millions of Westerners and engagingly chronicles Yogananda's search for enlightenment in India. He also describes his encounters with great figures such as Babaji, Anandamayi Ma, Mahatma Gandhi, and Rabindanath Tagore; his relationship with his beloved guru, Sri Yukteswar; and his eventual founding of the Self-Realization Fellowship in California. Yogananda freely discusses aspects of the science of yoga and the guru-disciple relationship that were previously kept secret. But what makes this book even more extraordinary is his honesty about the obstacles he faced along the way.

Radha: Story of a Woman's Search
by Swami Sivananda Radha

This extremely well-written, hard-to-put-down memoir is as much a portrait of Swami Sivananda and his Rishikesh ashram as it is about a woman's spiritual search and her experience on the path. Dancer Sylvia Hellman lived through two world wars in Germany and lost two husbands before immigrating to Canada in 1951. There, she joined a meditation group and immediately had a vision of Swami Sivananda. In 1955, at the age of 44, she gave up most of her possessions and undertook a rigorous trip to India to meet the great yogi, who embraced her as his spiritual daughter. She spent six months in intense study of yoga at his ashram. Time and again, she is filled with a Westerner's skepticism (such as why her guru does not look or act the way she expects him to), yet her misgivings are always allayed. At the end of her stay, Swami Sivananda initiated Radha as one of the first female swamis (against the wishes of many in his organization) and sent her home as a renunciate in a simple orange sari, with the mission of starting an ashram in Canada and bringing yoga to the West.

Autobiography of a Sadhu: A Journey into Mystic India
by Rampuri

"The real revolution is to transform yourself, not society. If you can succeed, then society will follow. The world is f—-d up, corrupted by capitalist elites, but we cannot hope to win any war on the material plane. Finding the Truth is the only way," writes Rampuri, the first foreigner to become a Nag Baba, India's order of naked, dreadlocked *sadhus* (renunciates) who live a nomadic life, follow Lord Shiva, and smear their bodies with ashes to stay warm. Born in Chicago and raised in Beverly Hills, Rampuri traveled to India in the 1960s at the age of 18. There, he met his guru, Hari Puri Baba, who instantly recognized him. Initiation followed, as did lessons in Hindi, Sanskrit, ayurveda, and mantra—and being an outsider. Rampuri experiences loads of fear, doubt, prejudice, and suffering along the way to full membership in what he calls the "Hell's Angels of Indian Spirituality," and eventually goes on to found his own ashram. Highly recommended for aspirants turned off by Westernized forms of yoga. (An earlier version of Rampuri's memoir is called *Baba: Autobiography of a Blue-Eyed Yogi.*)

The Journey Home: Autobiography of an American Swami
by Radhanath Swami

This entertaining chronicle of Richard "Monk" Slavin's transformation from questioning hippie to holy person is full of thrilling brush-with-death stories about his penniless overland journey across Europe and the Middle East to India in 1970. After arriving in India at the age of 19, the Chicago native meets a Who's Who of yogis, sadhus, and other holy people, including the Dalai Lama, Anandamayi Ma, S.N. Goenka, Swami Satchidananda, and Mother Teresa, and becomes a wandering monk who spends long periods of time in meditation. In this modern-day version of Paul Brunton's *A Search in Secret India*, he eventually commits to a guru, International Society for Krishna Consciousness founder Swami Prabhupada, and his path, Bhakti yoga. Now an international spiritual teacher, Radhanath Swami has founded a temple, a hospital, and an ashram in Maharashtra, India.

A Search in Secret India
by Paul Brunton

British-born Brunton traveled to India in the early 1930s in the hopes of encountering some real yogis. This thoroughly engaging classic text on the search for a guru by an excellent (albeit skeptical) writer provides a wonderful portrait of yogis, fakirs, and the fakers in Raj-era India. Brunton eventually finds and interviews the great master of *Jnana* yoga (yoga of wisdom), Sri Ramana Maharshi, who asks him repeatedly who is the *I* who is asking the questions, and tells him, "If you meditate on this question, Who am I?—if you begin to perceive that neither the body nor the brain nor the desires are really you, then the very attitude of enquiry will eventually draw the answer to you out of the depths of your own being; it will come to you of its own accord as a deep realization. Know the real self, and then the truth will shine forth within you like sunshine." Although he has two *samadhi* (enlightenment)-like experiences in his presence, Brunton leaves and resumes his search, eventually returning to Ramana Maharshi at the end of the book and asking to become his disciple.

My Guru and His Disciple
by Christopher Isherwood

This serious yet often funny book chronicles British writer Isherwood's 30-year relationship with his spiritual preceptor, Swami Prabhavananda, who opened the Vedanta Society of Southern California in 1930. Early on in the book, Isherwood, a great practitioner of *satya* (truthfulness), asks his future guru if he can lead a spiritual life while having a sexual relationship with a young man. "You must try to see him as the young Lord Krishna," says Prabhavananda. "From that point on, I began to understand that the Swami did not think in terms of sins, as most Christians do," writes Isherwood, who became deeply involved in the center and even considered becoming a monk and renouncing name and fame. Isherwood quotes liberally from his diaries, which gives the writing a visceral immediacy. Plus he's brutally honest about his own prejudices and spiritual stumbling blocks. (Isherwood and Prabhavananda co-wrote *How to Know God: The Yoga Aphorisms of Patanjali* and co-translated the *Bhagavad-Gita* and other texts; Isherwood also penned the excellent 1965 book *Ramakrishna and His Disciples*).

The Seven Storey Mountain: An Autobiography of Faith
by Thomas Merton

Christian mystic Thomas Merton's unblinking memoir about converting to Catholicism and becoming a Trappist monk is not directly about yoga, although his path is just like that of a yogi. My favorite moment in this gracefully written classic is when his friend Robert Lax asks him what his goal is, and Merton lamely replies that he wants to be a good Catholic. Lax retorts, "What you should say is that you want to be a saint." Flummoxed, Merton wrestles with the idea and says he cannot do it, thinking he cannot give up his sins and attachments. Lax replies, "All that is necessary to be a saint is to want to be one. Don't you believe that God will make you what He created you to be, if you will consent to let him do it? All you have to do is desire it." The next day, Merton tells his mentor, Mark Van Doren, "Lax is going around saying that all a man needs to be a saint is to want to be one." "Of course," his teacher replies.

Play of Consciousness: A Spiritual Autobiography
by Swami Muktananda

"Realization of God is only possible through a guru," writes Swami Muktananda in this 1978 bestseller. This sprawling memoir covers the time between Muktananda's spiritual initiation by Bhagavan Nityananda of Ganeshpuri in 1947 and his enlightenment nine years later. He is very specific yet matter-of-fact about his experiences in meditation and the visions he has along the way, which makes them seem all the more powerful. This is not an easy read—there's an assumption that the reader already understands many yogic concepts—but is an indispensable aid for students who are serious about Self-realization.

Further reading: Swami Ramdas, *In Quest of God: The Saga of an Extraordinary Pilgrimage*; Swami Rama, *Living with the Himalayan Masters*; Krishna Das, *Chants of a Lifetime*.

Part Four: Yoga Concepts

Part Four: Yoga Concepts

Yoga's Symbols, Sayings, and Sounds

From the ubiquitous *Om* to the 108 beads in the *mala* to *bandhas, chakras,* and *namaste,* there can be a lot of Sanskrit and symbolism in yoga. Here's a handy guide to some of the terms you may come across during your yoga journey.

Ahimsa
The first *yama* (ethical restraint) in yoga, ahimsa is nonharming of any living thing in word, thought, and deed. In class, students may practice ahimsa by not hurting themselves physically, verbally, or mentally.

Asana
Yoga posture. Defined in the *Yoga Sutras* as a steady, comfortable seat.

Atman
The individual Self or soul. According to nondualistic Vedanta philosophy, atman and Brahman (the Supreme Self) are one.

Bandha
A lock or energy seal used to control the *prana* (life force). The three main bandhas in *Hatha* yoga are *mula* bandha (contraction of the perineum), *uddiyana* bandha (contraction of the lower abdominal area), and *jalandhara* bandha (touching the chin to the chest).

Brahman

The Supreme Self or pure consciousness underlying Reality, according to Vedanta philosophy. Not to be confused with Brahma (the Hindu creator God) or *Brahmin* (the priestly caste).

Bhagavad-Gita

This yoga scripture is 18 chapters of the great Hindu epic *The Mahabharata*, but is often treated as a freestanding text. It is a battlefield discourse between Lord Krishna and his devotee, the warrior Arjuna, about *dharma*, the nature of the material and spiritual worlds, and the different paths of yoga. It contains the essence of the *Vedas* and is considered to be one of the world's most important literary and philosophical texts.

Chakras

The wheels or vortexes of energy in the *sushumna nadi* (major channel of energy in the subtle body). Each of the seven major chakras in the body corresponds to a major nerve plexus as well as to an organ or gland and a state of consciousness. The seven major chakra areas are: root, spleen, solar plexus, heart, throat, third eye, crown of head.

Dharma

Righteousness, order, law, virtue, correct behavior, duty, one's life purpose.

Disciple

A devotee or initiate of a guru who devotes his or her life to following and spreading the preceptor's teachings.

Guru

A spiritual preceptor. Literally, the remover of darkness.

Hatha Yoga

Hatha literally means sun ("ha") and moon ("tha"); it is the joining of the two opposites into a whole. Sometimes called the forceful path, hatha yoga uses bodily postures (asanas), breathing techniques (pranayama), and meditation (dhyana) to bring about radiant health, a calm mind and, ultimately, Self-realization. All of the practices that include asana, pranayama and meditation fall under the umbrella of hatha yoga.

Hatha Yoga Pradipika
The oldest of the three classic texts on Hatha yoga, compiled by Swami Svatmarama in the 15th century CE. It covers 15 asanas, as well as bandhas, *kriyas*, nadis, *mudras*, chakras, *pranayama*, and more.

Hindu deities
It is said that there are 30 crore (300 million) Hindu deities, each of which is thought to represent some aspect of the all-pervading Brahman, or cosmic consciousness. In yoga, the *ishta devata,* or chosen deity, is used as a tool of meditation and devotion until the consciousness merges with the deity, and it is no longer needed. Here are a few you may come across:

Ganesh, the elephant-headed god, the remover of obstacles and the son of Lord Shiva and Parvati. In *pujas* (ceremonies), he is worshipped first; he is also invoked before beginning a new enterprise.

The Hindu trimurti (three main forms of God) consists of Shiva, Vishnu, and Brahma. **Shiva** is the god of destruction and rebirth and is a favorite of yogis, as he is the supreme meditator and represents the innermost Self. The pose *natarajasana* (lord of the dance) is named for Lord Shiva's cosmic dance. **Vishnu** is the preserver, who incarnates and comes down to earth when dharma needs to be restored. **Lord Krishna** of the *Bhagavad-Gita* and **Lord Ram** from the *Ramayana* are avatars of Vishnu. **Brahma** is the creator, and should not to be confused with Brahmin (a caste), or Brahman (the formless god). Brahma is generally not worshipped (it's a long story), although there are a few temples devoted to him, including one in Rajasthan, India.

Hanuman is the monkey god who serves Lord Ram in the *Ramayanaya* and symbolizes devotion, courage, and loyalty. The name of the yoga pose *hanumanasana* (splits) comes from his great leap from India to Sri Lanka to bring Ram's ring to his kidnapped wife, **Sita,** who represents the ideal woman.

Parvati is the wife of Shiva and is the embodiment of divine female power. Two of her avatars are **Kali,** the compassionate and protective goddess of destruction and rebirth who destroys the lower nature, and the warrior goddess **Durga.**

Lakshmi is the wife of Vishnu and represents spiritual and material prosperity.

Saraswati, the consort of Brahma and the sister of Lakshmi, is the goddess of music, the arts, and education. She is considered the mother of the *Vedas* (the oldest scriptures of Hinduism).

NOTE: It is offensive to many people to see images of these gods on feet, shoes, pants, yoga mats or rugs, etc.

Karma
Literally, action, but it implies destiny or fate. For every action, there is a reaction. If you commit a selfish action, you will eventually have to pay the price. There are three types of karma: *sanchita* (accumulated), *prarabdha* (the karma we are dealing with in this lifetime, which was generated in a previous lifetime), and *agami* (karma we are creating in this lifetime).

Kirtan
Call-and-response devotional chanting that is part of the *Bhakti* (devotional) yoga path.

Kleshas
Colorings, obstacles, impurities, mental patterns, defects, or afflictions of the mind that are the cause of pain and suffering. They are *avidya* (ignoring the Real Self), *asmita* (egoism), *raga* (attachment), *dvesha* (aversion), and *abhinivesha* (clinging to life).

Koshas
The five sheaths or coverings that obscure the atman, one's inmost Self, in Vedanta philosophy. They are *annamaya* kosha (physical/body sheath), *pranamaya* kosha (energy sheath), *manamaya* kosha (lower mind sheath), *vijnanamaya* kosha (higher mind or wisdom sheath), and *anandamaya* kosha (bliss sheath).

Kriya
Cleansing practice. Use of the neti pot, a device used for irrigating nasal passages, is a type of kriya.

Mala
A beaded rosary that is used to count oral or mental repetitions of a *mantra*. This practice is called *japa*, which is a meditation tool and an effective way to calm the mind. A mala often has 108 beads (a sacred number in Hinduism and other traditions) plus a center "guru" bead. Specific ways to handle and use the mala can differ from lineage to lineage.

Mantra
A Sanskrit sound, syllable, word, or phrase that can be used for spiritual advancement. Each sound in Sanskrit creates a vibration that is thought to produce a special effect on the gross and subtle body and mind, so correct pronunciation is important. There is a mantra for every occasion; the simplest mantra is "Om." (See "Mantra and Japa" for a list of other mantras).

Maya
Illusion—or the idea that what we can perceive through the senses is the only reality.

Mudra
A gesture, seal, or hand position that guides the prana. A widely practiced mudra is *Jnana* **mudra**: the gesture or seal of knowledge representing the enlightened state, often used during pranayama and meditation. In many traditions, the tip of the forefinger (representing the ego) touches the tip of the thumb (representing the true Self), creating a perfect circle with no beginning or end.

Nadis
The 72,000 subtle energy channels through which prana flows. One of the goals of Hatha yoga is to remove blockages in the nadis so that prana can flow and the *jiva* (individual) can experience the

Supreme Self. The three main nadis are the *shoshumna* (center), *ida* (left), and *pingala* (right).

Namaste
Often said at the end of a yoga class with palms in prayer at the front of the chest, namaste is considered an informal greeting or salutation in India, where it's a shortened version of *namaskar* (which literally means "I bow to your form"). It is usually not said at the end of class in traditional systems. In the West, namaste has sometimes come to mean "The divinity in me bows to the divinity in you."

Om or Aum (pranava)
Om is perhaps the most common sound and symbol one comes across in yoga class—and the most sacred. Om is considered to be the primeval sound, the sound of the universe, the sound from which all other sounds are formed. "The cosmic sound of Om contains all the 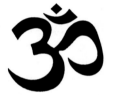 names, all the forms of the Divine," says Swami Sivananda Radha in her book *Time to Be Holy*. The yoga scriptures state that there is no difference between the sound "Om" and God, the Supreme Consciousness.

Om has three syllables: ahh, ooo (as in "oh," with the mouth shaped like an "o"), and mmm. It is often followed by silence, in which to feel the vibration and effect of the sound.

In the symbol for Om, the dot on top represents the real Self. The top curve represents *maya*, or illusion. The other curves represent the three states: deep sleep, the dream state, and the waking state.

NOTE: Many people find it offensive to see the sacred Om symbol on feet, shoes, pants, yoga mats and rugs, etc.

Prana
The vital life force; said to be contained in the breath.

Pranayama
Control of the prana (breath). Pranayama should be learned under the guidance of a guru or qualified teacher.

Purusha, Prakriti, and the Gunas
Purusha is Pure Consciousness; prakriti is matter or nature. Prakriti consists of the three gunas: *sattva* (harmony), *rajas* (action) and *tamas* (inertia), which are always at play. Becoming a witness of the gunas and not identifying with them can bring one closer to purusha.

Samadhi
Oneness. Samadhi is the goal of yoga, and is the non-dualistic state of consciousness in which one merges with the object of concentration and loses all thoughts of separateness.

Shanti or Shanthi
Peace. The correct pronunciation is with emphasis on the first syllable: "SHAHN-tee," not "shahn-TEE." It is often chanted three times at the end of a mantra or yoga class— for peace in body, speech, and mind—or as a wish for peace of mind within the self, with others, and with the environment. (If shanti is repeated three times, the final one is often pronounced "Shan-TIH-hee.").

Tapas
Literally, heat. The third *Niyama* (observance) in *Raja* (royal) yoga; austerities or practices of self-discipline that purify body and mind so the Self can be realized.

Yoga
To yoke or reunite with God or the Supreme Self, and the method through which this is achieved. There are several paths of yoga, including Hatha yoga (postures, breathing and meditation), *Bhakti* yoga (the yoga of devotion), *Karma* yoga (the yoga of selfless service), and Jnana yoga (the yoga of knowledge). In the West, the word *yoga* is often used to refer to the postures or asanas of Hatha yoga.

Yoga Sutras of Patanjali

Its four chapters and 196 aphorisms outline the path of Raja yoga or control of the mind—one of the six orthodox schools of Hindu philosophy. It comprises the definition of yoga (the cessation of the fluctuations of the mind) as well as the eight limbs (*ashtanga*) of yoga, including its ethical roots (the *yamas*). Patanjali, who codified and recorded the *Yoga Sutras*, is considered to be an incarnation of Lord Vishnu's serpent, Adishesha.

Yogi

One who practices yoga. "Anyone who practices a scientific technique for divine realization is a yogi," writes Paramahansa Yogananda in *Autobiography of a Yogi*.

The Eight Limbs of Yoga

Compiled by the sage Patanjali Maharishi in the *Yoga Sutras*, the eight limbs are a series of steps or disciplines that purify the body and mind, ultimately leading the yogi to enlightenment. Also called *Ashtanga* yoga, these eight limbs are the foundation of *Raja* (royal) yoga:

Yama—restraints or "don'ts"
Niyama—observances of self-discipline or "dos"
Asana—physical postures (literally, a steady, comfortable seat)
Pranayama—control of the breath or *prana* (energy)
Pratyahara—withdrawal or control of the senses
Dharana—concentration
Dhyana—meditation, or complete absorption into the object of meditation
Samadhi—the super-conscious state in which nonduality is experienced; the deepest and highest state of consciousness where body and mind have been transcended and the yogi is established in Oneness with the Self or God

The yamas and niyamas are the ethical underpinnings of yoga and are practiced in conjunction with asana. They each are divided into five moral injunctions, aimed at taming the lower nature. The yamas and niyamas should be practiced in word, thought, and deed, regardless of time, place, and circumstance.

The yamas:
Ahimsa—nonharming of both the self and other living creatures in word, thought, and deed
Satya—truthfulness; being true to others and ourselves

Asteya—nonstealing; controlling the desire for power, objects, or undeserved credit (if you are established in asteya, all wealth will come to you)

Brahmacharya—continence, or moderation in all things, including diet; celibacy; practice of brahmacharya results in tremendous energy and willpower

Aparigraha—noncovetousness, nonhoarding, the elimination of greed; bestows peace, contentment, satisfaction, and fearlessness

The niyamas:

Saucha—purity, or internal and external cleanliness; includes the mind (which must be freed from feelings of lust, envy, pride, fear, jealousy, arrogance, hatred, and delusion); can be aided by use of *mantra* (repetition of a sacred word or phrase), *kirtan* (call-and-response chanting), reading of holy texts, and association with holy people

Santosha—contentment; desirelessness; being grateful for what you have.

Tapas—purifying austerity, self-discipline/control; can include intense asana practice

Svadhyaya—Self-study, which includes reading spiritual texts and contemplation

Ishwara pranidhana—relinquishing the ego, or living with a constant awareness of one's true nature; surrender to God's will

The Four Main Paths of Yoga

"The Yoga of synthesis alone is suitable for this modern age.
The four yogas are interdependent and inseparable. Love is
endowed in service. Service is love in expression. Knowledge is
diffused love and love is concentrated knowledge. Karma Yoga
is always combined with Bhakti Yoga and Jnana Yoga. Bhakti Yoga
is the fulfillment of Karma Yoga. Raja Yoga is the fulfillment
of Karma Yoga and Bhakti Yoga. Jnana Yoga is the fulfillment
of Karma Yoga, Bhakti Yoga and Raja Yoga."
—Swami Sivananda

Many of us come to yoga through the practice of *asana* (yoga poses). While asana gives us radiant health, it is just one part of a complete yoga practice—the goal of which is union with the spark of the divine residing within all living beings.

There are four main paths of yoga: *Raja* (royal), *Bhakti* (devotion), *Karma* (work or action), and *Jnana* (knowledge).

When considering a primary path, choose the one that is most pleasant. My *param-guru* (my guru's spiritual preceptor), Swami Kailashananda, said to do all of the practices, but to focus on the path that suits your tendencies.

Raja yoga: the science of physical and mental control

Literally, the royal path of yoga, Raja is the yoga of mind and body control. Its focus is to turn mental and physical energy into spiritual energy.

The roadmap for the practice is the eight limbs of yoga (*Ashtanga* yoga), as outlined in the *Yoga Sutras* of Patanjali. Asana and *pranayama* (breathing) are considered a subset of Raja yoga known as *Hatha* yoga.

The eight limbs are *yama* (nonharming, truthfulness, non-stealing, celibacy, nongreed), *niyama* (internal and external purity, contentment, austerity, self-study, and surrender of the ego), asana (postures; literally, "a steady, comfortable seat"), pranayama, *pratyahara* (withdrawal of the senses), *dharana* (concentration), *dhyana* (meditation), and *samadhi* (union with the divine).

In Raja yoga, one begins with the gross and works towards the subtle. Before controlling the mind, one learns to control one's actions and body, then the breath, the senses, and, finally, the mind.

The practice: The Raja yogi should try to practice the ethical roots (yama and niyama) at all times. Sri Dharma Mittra says, "Without yama, there is no yoga." If you can only practice one of the ethical roots, the most important is *ahimsa* (nonharming, which includes not eating animals). The ultimate Raja yoga practice consists of meditation, but it can also include asana, breathing, *bandhas* (internal bonds or locks), relaxation, *mudras* (gestures), and the ethical roots to control the body and move the *prana* (subtle life force) up the spine.

Ideal for: everyone, including athletes, intellectuals, multi-taskers, and those who possess a mystical nature.

Resources
How to Know God: The Yoga Aphorisms of Patanjali
    by Swami Prabhavananda and Christopher Isherwood
The *Yoga Sutras of Patanjali* by Swami Satchidananda
The *Yoga Sutras of Patanjali* by Dr. Edwin Bryant
The *Hatha Yoga Pradipika* by Brian Dana Akers

Karma yoga: the yoga of action or selfless service
Swami Sivananda said, "Feel that you are an instrument in the hands of the Lord. Feel that the Lord works through your body, mind and senses. Offer all your actions to the Lord. Offer the fruits of your actions to the Lord. This is the way to do self-surrender."

Karma yoga is selfless service. The *Bhagavad-Gita* explains, "To work, alone, you are entitled, never to its fruit. Neither let your motive be the fruit of action, nor let your attachment be to non-action" (II.47).

This practice quickly dissolves the ego, which yogis believe separates us from our true nature of pure bliss, peace, and knowledge.

Although volunteer work is the most obvious form of Karma yoga, every type of work can be turned into selfless service if one renounces the fruits and fixes the mind on the Supreme Goal.

As Swami Vishnudevananda explained, "Karma Yoga is not simply action. It is removing the idea of agency, the thought, 'I am the doer.' That must go. You are not the doer. We are not the doer. Within all action, there is infinite power, God's power working. Can you see? That power makes this body move. Karma Yoga removes the egoism, 'I am the doer.'"

The practice: Volunteer to help the poor or sick or your spiritual preceptor, and assist others in small ways whenever possible. Before doing asana (or performing any action), set your intention and offer it to the Supreme Self, chosen deity, or something equally unselfish. For daily tasks, say a prayer or recite a *mantra* (repetition of God's name) while working. Every action can be considered Karma yoga if it is done selflessly. Ideally, Karma yoga is practiced anonymously (i.e., don't brag about it or put it in your bio or on your Facebook page; do it simply because it has to be done).

Ideal for: Everyone, especially extraverts; workaholics; those who are interested in social justice; or those who struggle with ego, selfishness, anxiety, or depression.

Resources
The *Bhagavad-Gita* (Swami Nikhilananda)
Karma Yoga by Swami Vivekananda
Practice of Karma Yoga by Swami Sivananda
Volunteer opportunities: volunteermatch.org or idealist.org

Bhakti yoga: the path of devotion or divine love
Swami Kailashananda said, "Devotion to God is total surrender of the ego." Bhakti yoga is devotion to or love of God; all love and emotions for worldly things are channeled into love for the divine. It is considered the easiest path.

According to the *Vishnu Purana (Srimad Bhagavata)* (7.5.23-24), there are nine forms of bhakti: *sravana* (hearing stories of God), *kirtan* (singing of God's glories), *smarana* (remembrance of

His name and presence), *padasevana* (service), *archana* (worship of an image), *vandana* (prostration to the Lord), *dasya* (servitude), *sakhya* (friendship), and *atmanivedana* (complete surrender of the self).

Swami Sivananda said, "The Bhakti Yogi is motivated chiefly by the power of love and sees God as the embodiment of love. Through prayer, worship and ritual he surrenders himself to God, channeling and transmuting his emotions into unconditional love or devotion. Chanting or singing the praises of God form a substantial part of Bhakti Yoga."

The practice: It is helpful to have an *ishta devata* (chosen deity) from one's personal religious faith or elsewhere. The devotee may relate to God in the way that is most natural to him or her, much as he/she would relate to a parent, lover, friend, or child. Practice can include reading stories, worship, or visiting holy places. Mantra and kirtan are two of the most accessible Bhakti practices. Many yoga studios offer kirtan.

Ideal for: Those who are passionate or emotional or have an innately devotional nature.

Resources
The *Bhagavad-Gita* (Swami Nikhilananda)
Bhagavata Purana (Srimad Bhagavatam)
   translated by Kamala Subramaniam
Bhakti-Yoga: The Yoga of Love and Devotion by Swami Vivekananda
The Practice of Bhakti Yoga by Swami Sivananda

Jnana yoga: the yoga of knowledge
Adi Sankaracharya said, "God only is real. The world is unreal. The individual is none other than God." Jnana means knowledge of Brahman (Supreme Self) and *atman* (individual soul), and the realization of their unity. Called the most direct and difficult path, Jnana yoga is most suitable for those with strong willpower and intellect. One inquires again and again into the nature of the mind, and strives to go beyond it to the inner witness or Supreme Self that observes all and is one with all. Contemplation of the *koshas* (the five sheaths surrounding the atman, or inmost self) eventually leads one to the atman.

The doctrine of the Jnani is *"neti, neti "* ("not this, not this"), popularized by the great Jnani Sri Ramana Maharshi as a way to discriminate between the indescribable imperishable Brahman (God without attributes) and what is not Brahman. In other words, one realizes one is not their body, mind, or senses, but is something greater: the pure, undivided consciousness that pervades everything. As Sri Dharma Mittra says, "If you can see it, it's not you."

Ramana Maharshi said, "But it does not mean exactly discarding of the non-Self, it means the finding of the real Self. The real Self is the infinite 'I'. That 'I' is perfection. It is eternal. It has no origin and no end. The other 'I' is born and also dies. It is impermanent. See to whom the changing thoughts belong. They will be found to arise after the 'I'-thought. Hold the 'I'-thought and they subside. Trace back the source of the 'I'-thought. The Self alone will remain."

Sometimes called *vedanta*, this path is greatly aided by practice of the other three. As the Sivananda Yoga Vedanta Center explains on its website, "Before practicing Jnana yoga, the aspirant needs to have integrated the lessons of the other yogic paths, for without selflessness and love of God, strength of body and mind, the search for Self-realization can become mere idle speculation."

The practice: Contemplate what is behind the five koshas or sheaths: *annamaya* kosha (physical), *pranamaya* kosha (energy), *manamaya* kosha (lower mind), *vijnanamaya* kosha (higher mind), and *anandamaya* kosha (bliss). Practice neti, neti and discriminate between what is always changing and what is not subject to time, space, and causation. With the help of a qualified teacher, read and contemplate the main Jnana scriptures. After contemplation comes Self-Knowledge and then, finally, realization.

Ideal for: Intellectuals, introverts, and atheists.

Resources
Self-Knowledge: Atma Bodha (Swami Nikhilananda)
Talks on Sankara's Vivekachoodamani by Swami Chinmayananda
The *Upanishads* (Swami Nikhilananda)
Talks with Sri Ramana Maharshi
I Am That: Talks with Sri Nisargadatta Maharaj

Yoga Scripture: The Primary Texts

Many of us are introduced to yoga through the postures, or *asanas.* But the asanas are just one small component in the larger system of yoga, wherein the goal is Self-realization, or union with the divine.

A handful of scriptural texts explain the philosophy behind this larger yoga system, which is actually several paths that lead to the same place. Each path, like each text, is suited to a different temperament (see "The Four Main Paths of Yoga").

Text: The *Dhammapada*
Path: Theravada Buddhism (which touches on all four main paths of yoga)
Overview: While technically not a yoga text, this lyrical collection of the Buddha's teachings encompasses many yogic ideas in a simple, nondogmatic form that is easy to grasp for beginners and those who are averse to the terms *God* and *scripture*. It includes many teachings from yoga philosophy, including mind control, karma and reincarnation, nonviolence, nonattachment, right conduct, concentrating the mind, cultivating wisdom, and surrendering the ego.
Core Teaching: We are each responsible for our own situation; with self-effort and self-control, anyone can achieve lasting peace and contentment.
Key Quote: "Come, look on this world / As a beautiful royal chariot. / Fools flounder in it, / But the discerning do not cling."
Bonus Fact: My guru, Sri Dharma Mittra, recommends *The Dhammapada* for beginners on the yoga path.

Recommended Translation: Gil Fronsdal's 2005 book and audio CD set published by Shambhala, which includes a recording of the text read by venerable Buddhist teacher Jack Kornfield.

Text: The *Yoga Sutras of Patanjali*

Path: *Raja* yoga, or the royal path of yoga: the yoga of mind control

Overview: The sage Patanjali codified these ancient teachings in the second century BCE, and their four parts define yoga and explain how it is to be practiced and achieved as well as obstacles and distractions on the path. These *sutras,* or threads, outline the foundational eight limbs of yoga and such terms as the *yamas* (ethical roots), *kleshas* (obstacles), and *gunas* (qualities of the material world); there are also clear explanations of different meditation practices and their benefits.

Core Teaching: Only a controlled mind can achieve infinite bliss and peace.

Key Quote: *Yogash chitta vritti nirodhah.* ("Yoga is the cessation of the thought-currents of the mind.")

Bonus Fact: Patanjali is said to be an incarnation of Adishesha (Lord Vishnu's serpent), who is in turn one of the many incarnations of Lord Vishnu, the preserver of the universe.

Recommended Translations: *How to Know God: The Yoga Aphorisms of Patanjali* by Swami Prabhavananda and Christopher Isherwood; *The Yoga Sutras of Patanajali* by Swami Satchidananda; *The Yoga Sutras of Patañjali: A New Edition, Translation, and Commentary* by Edwin F. Bryant Adwaita Das; *Light on the Yoga Sutras of Patanjali* by BKS Iyengar.

Text: The *Hatha Yoga Pradipika*

Path: *Hatha* yoga (the yoga of union), which includes postures, breathing, and cleansing practices

Overview: *Hatha* means sun-moon, or willful or forceful, and *pradipika* means to throw light on; the goal of Hatha yoga is to unite *prana* and *apana* (the upward and downward-moving energies). This manual was codified by Swami Svatarama in the 15th century CE, although the practices have been around much longer. Its four chapters provide instructions on postures, breathing, *bandhas* (energy seals), *kriyas* (cleansing practices), and *mudras* (gestures) designed to awaken the *kundalini* (latent cosmic energy) as well as information on the subtle body; the 15 postures it outlines include *simhasana* (lion pose), *mayurasana* (peacock pose) and *kurmasana* (tortoise pose).

Core Teaching: Raja yoga is not possible without Hatha yoga, and vice-versa.

Key Quote: "The yogi perishes by six causes: over-eating, hard physical labor, too much talk, the observance of [unsuitable] vows, promiscuous company, and unsteadiness. The yogi succeeds by six qualifications: cheerfulness, perseverance, courage, true knowledge, firm belief in the words of the guru, and by abandoning unsuitable company."

Bonus Facts: The other two classic texts on Hatha yoga are the *Gheranda Samhita* and the *Shiva Samhita*. Three excellent modern companion books are BKS Iyengar's *Light on Yoga*, Swami Vishnudevananda's *The Complete Illustrated Book of Yoga*, and Dharma Mittra's *Asanas: 608 Yoga Poses*.

Recommended Translations: Those by Brian Dana Akers, Swami Vishnudevananda, Swami Muktibodhananda Saraswati, and Pancham Sinh (the last contains very little commentary).

Text: The *Bhagavad-Gita*

Path: Karma and Bhakti yoga (also Jnana yoga and Raja yoga)

Overview: This 700-verse "Song of God" is part of the larger Hindu epic the *Mahabharata*, which dates from between the fifth and second centuries BCE and is attributed to the sage Vyasa. Set on the battlefield as a conversation between the warrior Arjuna and Lord Krishna, its eighteen chapters are considered a primary text on the major paths of yoga. Its poetic verses explain karma and reincarnation, the nature of the soul, the gunas and *dharma* (life's purpose); this is an indispensable text for anyone who is serious about Self-realization.

Core Teaching: A yogi is entitled to work, but never to its result.

Key Quote: "He is said to be a steadfast yogi whose heart, through knowledge and realization, is filled with satisfaction, who, having conquered his senses, never vacillates, and to whom a clod, a stone, and gold are the same."

Bonus Fact: Mahatma Gandhi referred to the *Gita* as a "spiritual dictionary" and found great solace in it, particularly in the last nineteen verses of Chapter II.

Recommended Translations: Swami Nikhilananda's translations (one with commentary and one without) are lyrical yet straightforward. Beginners may prefer Eknath Easwaran's three-part translation, which includes protracted commentary. Swami Satchidananda's *The Living Gita* is also suitable for beginners.

Text: *Srimad Bhagavatam or Bhagavata Purana (Divine Eternal Tales of Supreme God)*

Path: Bhakti yoga (the path of devotion)

Overview: This engaging collection of tales of the Hindu gods and sages focuses on the incarnations of Lord Vishnu, the preserver, particularly in the form of Krishna. Passed down orally through the centuries, these tales were codified by the sage Vyasa in the sixth or ninth century CE. The chapters on Lord Krishna detail the nine practices of Bhakti yoga, one of which is to read and hear the songs of *the Bhagavatam*. The lengthy text also contains instruction on Jnana and Karma yoga.

Core Teaching: One can achieve liberation through cultivating a personal relationship with Lord Vishnu via His form as Krishna.

Key Quote: "If one always chants the holy name of the Lord with great devotion in the evening and in the morning, one can become free from all material miseries."

Bonus Fact: Many of the stories and dramas found in popular culture can be traced back to this text.

Recommended Translation: Kamala Subramaniam's 2006 translation.

Text: The *Upanishads*

Path: Jnana yoga (the path of knowledge or wisdom)

Overview: The *Upanishads* are the foundation of the path of wisdom, or *vedanta*, the rigorous nondual path that is suitable for those with strong willpower and intellect. *Upanishad* means "sitting close to" and traditionally the *Upanishads*—the concluding portion of the *Vedas*—were learned directly from a Self-realized teacher in a pastoral setting. There are 200 *Upanishads*, of which 13 are considered principal. They describe the nature of the Supreme Self and explore the yogic concepts of karma and reincarnation, *moksha* (liberation), *atman,* and *nirguna Brahman* (God without attributes) as well as the nature of Om and how to meditate on it.

Core Teachings: Brahman (the Supreme Self or Cosmic Consciousness) and atman (the individual soul) are one and the same; everything perceived through the senses is a construction of the mind.

Key Quote: *Tat Tvam Asi.* ("Thou art That / That thou art.")

Bonus Fact: Scholars have noted similarities between ideas contained in the *Upanishads,* some of which date back to 800 to 400 BCE, and the writings of Plato and Kant.

Side Note: It is advisable to be established in yama and *niyama* (yoga's ethical roots) and firmly grounded in the teachings of the *Yoga Sutras,* the *Bhagavad-Gita,* and Adi Shankaracharya's *Self-Knowledge* before approaching the *Upanishads.* Having a guru as a guide is essential.

Recommended Translation: Swami Nikhilananda's four-volume set.

How to read scripture

Many yogis begin with the *Yoga Sutras,* and then move on to the *Bhagavad-Gita* and *Hatha Yoga Pradipika.*

When deciding on a translation, choose one with commentary that resonates with you. You will find that your preference will change as your consciousness evolves. Eventually, you will be able to read and understand scripture without commentary. At that stage, it is helpful to read one sutra or stanza or *sloka* (Sanskrit verse) at a time, and contemplate it before moving on. Scripture is meant to be read and re-read, and it can take years to master a single chapter or passage, let alone an entire work.

Traditionally, scripture is treated with respect. Accordingly, have clean hands and refrain from eating or drinking while reading. Also, such texts should not to be placed on the floor or a bed or near/on shoes. It should not be read in bed or taken into the bathroom.

When reading, sit tall with a straight spine. You might wish to wear a prayer shawl.

Guidance from a guru or qualified teacher is critical when reading scripture. As Geetha Iyengar once told *Yoga Journal,* "It is only after a student has been shown a method by a guru and is totally involved on a yogic path that the real meaning of Patanjali's *Yoga Sutra* will reveal itself."

Om, the Sacred Pranava

"Brahman is Om, this whole world is Om."
—*Taittiriya Upanishad*

Mispronounced, misunderstood, and misconstrued, the sacred *Om*, or *Aum*, is the root of all mantras and contains all the sounds in the world. Yogis believe the Om is one and the same as Brahman, or the ultimate reality underlying the phenomenal world.

deep, dreamless sleep / turiya / maya / dreaming / waking

But sometimes the meaning—and pronunciation—can get lost. A couple of years ago, I was waiting for a large class to end in the room where I was about to teach a workshop. They finally finished with three loud, wall-shaking "Ums." Not the "Om" that rhymes with "home," but "Um," which rhymes with "thumb."

The Om and all the mantras that spring from it are like *asanas* (yoga postures) for the mouth and should be pronounced with care and concentration as well as with proper motivation, faith, devotion, and understanding. In the scriptures, Om is also referred to as the *pranava, omkara,* or *udgita.*

According to yogis, the sound and form of Om is the same as God. The *Rig Veda* says, "In the beginning was Brahman, with whom was the Word, and the Word was truly the supreme Brahman." The *Bible* says something similar: "In the beginning was the Word" and "The Word was with God, and the Word was God."

Most mantras begin and end with Om; it is the highest of all mantras or divine words, as well as Brahman itself. In the

Bhagavad-Gita, Lord Krishna says to Arjuna, "I am the father of this universe, the mother, the support and the grandsire. I am the object of knowledge, the purifier and the syllable Om. I am also the *Rig,* the *Sama* and the *Yajur Vedas.*"

The *Yoga Sutras* of Patanjali states that the Om is *Isvara,* or God: "The sacred word designating this creative source is the sound OM, called Pranava. This sound is remembered with deep feeling for the meaning of what it represents. From that remembering comes the realization of the individual Self and the removal of obstacles."

Because the Om is considered to be one and the same as God by many yogis and Hindus, it should be treated with respect. Consequently, having it tattooed on the foot or ankle or printed on a pant leg or across the buttocks or on shoes or a yoga mat (where the feet step on it) or placing the Om symbol on the floor are considered highly disrespectful. Knowingly offending others in this way is a violation of *ahimsa,* or nonharming.

The Om has four parts. The first is the "A," which sounds like the "a" in father and is pronounced in the throat, with the mouth wide open. It is usually fairly short. The second is the long, loud "u," which rhymes with home and is pronounced with the mouth actively shaped like an "o"—not with a slack mouth. The sound rolls over the tongue. Then the mouth slowly closes and the sound becomes the "m," which is pronounced "mmmm" with the lips together, creating a pleasant vibration. The fourth is the silence that follows. My guru, Sri Dharma Mittra, says that during the silence one should focus on the vibration behind the forehead.

The three parts of the Om represent the three states in the manifest world: the "A" is the waking state (represented by the bottom curve of the Om symbol), the "u" is the dreaming state (the middle curve), and the "m" is the state of deep, dreamless sleep (the top curve). The silence that follows represents the fourth state or *turiya*—the pure consciousness that pervades and illumines the other three states. It is represented by the *bindu,* or dot, at the top, while the curve separating it from the rest of the Om symbolizes *maya,* or illusion.

The Om also relates to the three bodies: the "A" is the gross body, the "u" is the subtle body, and the "m" represents the causal body. It also contains the three *gunas,* or qualities of the phenomenal world that are constantly shifting: "A" is *rajas* (action), "u" is *sattva* (harmony), and "m" is *tamas* (inertia). Finally, Om represents the Hindu trinity: the "A" is creation, or *Brahma,* the "u" is preservation or Vishnu, and "m" is dissolution, or Lord Shiva.

Some yogis believe that what you are thinking of when you die is where you will go next. So if you only learn one mantra in this lifetime, let it be the Om, which represents the supreme goal. If Om is always on your lips when you are alive, it will be in your mind when you pass.

As the *Bhagavad-Gita* says, "He who closes all the doors to the senses, confines the mind within the heart, draws the prana into the head, and engages in the practice of yoga, uttering Om, the single syllable denoting Brahman, and meditates on Me—he who so departs, leaving the body, attains the Supreme Goal."

Om meditation

There are many Om meditations. This one, which I learned directly from Sri Dharma Mittra, is suitable for all levels.

Face east or north. Sit tall on the floor or a chair, with the back of the neck in line with the spine. Inhale, then exhale, creating a long, loud, resonant Om. The mouth is wide open during the "A"; in the shape of an "o" during the "u"; with the lips coming together for the "m," which should last for at least one-third of the Om. Then remain silent and mentally "say" Om while focusing on the vibration between the eyebrows and behind the forehead. Then repeat: a verbal Om, followed by a mental Om. Keep repeating for ten minutes. This practice stimulates the pituitary gland, activates the sixth sense, and is an antidote to depression.

ॐ *Part Four: Yoga Concepts*

The Guru-Disciple Relationship

"You need an external guru as a means to attain the guru within you. Sometimes you may become egotistical and decide, 'I don't need a guru.' That is the ego talking. You must tame it."
—Swami Rama

It is said that three of the highest blessings on the spiritual path are a human birth, finding a true guru, and receiving initiation from the guru.

A yoga teacher can share amazing asana sequences, alignment tips, and other practices that help the student to achieve radiant health, improve his or her conduct, and feel really, really good.

But it is said that only a guru can bring the student face to face with God.

"There is no more powerful way of overcoming the vicious nature and old samskaras [tendencies] in the aspirants than personal contact with and service to the Guru," said Swami Sivananda. "Guru's Grace will, in a mysterious manner, enable the disciples to perceive the spiritual power within, though it is impossible for the Guru to point out God or Brahman to be this or that."

Guru means dispeller of darkness, and in the yoga tradition, spiritual knowledge is transmitted directly from guru to disciple, a practice dating back millennia to the time of the ancient *rishis* (seers). It is believed that the goal of Self-realization cannot be reached without the help of the guru, or spiritual preceptor, who has already reached the goal and knows how to safely guide others to it. Some of the greatest yogis, such as Paramahansa Yogananda, Adi Shankaracharya, and Sri Ramakrishna, all had gurus. Even Jesus had John the Baptist.

The teacher can only bring the student as far along the path as he or she has personally traveled. If one's yoga goal is Self-realization, then a Self-realized guru or preceptor is absolutely necessary.

"The role of Guru is of the highest importance, as is the sincerity, humility, and loyalty of the student," says my guru, Sri Dharma Mittra. "His grace enables the disciple to perceive the latent spiritual power within, and shows the doorway to the Super-consciousness," he continues. "But it is the disciple who must step through it."

"Many students, according to their own fancy, select their own method of *sadhana* [practice] without considering the consequences," said Swami Sivananda. "Improper diet, wrong sadhana without a proper guide, hard and foolish austerities on a weak body, torturing the body in the name of *tapasya* [austerities], have entirely ruined many aspirants. Therefore a personal Guru is necessary to give timely instructions according to the change of seasons, circumstances and progress."

How does one know who is a true guru? The guru is often the humblest person in the room; she is the first to help and the last to be served. The guru is like a manifestation of God, embodying love and compassion and the qualities of the yogi as described in the scriptures; he/she is steeped in *sattva* (peace or harmony). The guru can also be a strict disciplinarian, but his or her actions are always guided by selfless love.

When Swami Vishnudevananda met Swami Sivananda for the second time, he was either too timid or too arrogant to bow down to him; so Swami Sivananda humbly prostrated fully before Swami Vishnudevananda, completely disarming him.

In *Be Love Now: The Path of the Heart*, Ram Dass writes, "Someone asked Maharaj-ji [Neem Karoli Baba], 'How do I know if someone is my guru?' Maharaj-ji said, 'Do you think s/he can fulfill you in every way spiritually? Do you feel s/he can free you from all desires and attachments? Do you feel s/he can lead you to final liberation?'"

The guru-disciple relationship can be formalized and cemented by *mantra* (sacred word) initiation, in which the guru gives the disciple a specifically chosen mantra. The mantra creates a psychic link to the guru; the more often and sincerely the disciple repeats the mantra, the stronger the bond. (Sri Dharma says that spiritual knowledge can only be transmitted psychically.) The disciple may be given a new name to help him or her shed the past and old ego-identity. The name symbolizes a rebirth in consciousness; Yogi Bhajan likened it to a prayer that calls us back to our true Self.

Mantra initiation is not a casual undertaking. It creates a bond more lasting and sacred than marriage; the guru does everything possible to guide the disciple's spiritual growth. But the disciple must do the work. It is said that if the disciple does not reach the goal in this lifetime, the guru must be reborn along with the disciple so they can go through the whole process again. The pattern is repeated until the aspirant achieves Self-realization. No sincere aspirant wants to be responsible for the guru undergoing another birth.

The guru may recognize the disciple. But the impetus is entirely on the aspirant to find the guru and to make sure the guru is worthy. The preceptor's actions should be unselfish and embody the teachings of yoga. The aspirant should study and even test the preceptor carefully before becoming a disciple. That's what the future Swami Vivekananda did when he secretly hid a coin under Sri Ramakrishna's mattress. When Ramakrishna came in and sat down on the bed, he immediately jumped up as if he'd been stung.

Sri Ramakrishna encouraged his disciples to question him. "Test me as the money-changer tests coins," he said. "Before you decide to accept a guru, watch him by day and night."

The guru may also test the disciple, of course. Sri Ramakrishna tested Swami Vivekananda many times.

For most aspirants, a living guru is a must; that way the ego does not get in the way, and there are no doubts about the instructions. The aspirant should stick to one guru for the same reason. Jumping from preceptor to preceptor will only cause confusion and doubt.

My guru often says that yoga is "total obedience to the teacher," which is another reason to study the guru before making a commitment. (The only exception to the "total obedience" rule is if the instruction goes against the disciple's conscience. Not against the ego, which must be thinned to reach the goal, but against the conscience.) A good disciple should be loyal and reverent and ever ready to serve the guru.

Dharma Mittra says, "The student who is under the guidance of Guru is safe from all. Guru is your fortress against your lower nature and all obstacles and difficulties. But you must follow the Guru's guidance implicitly."

Nothing pleases the guru more than seeing the disciple stand on his or her own two feet; at some point the disciple must do the practices taught by the guru alone and eventually experience the Supreme Truth. The sequence is to find the guru, love the guru, and then leave the guru.

"I am always ready to help you," said Swami Sivananda. "My sympathies are ever with you. I will radiate joy, peace, and thought-currents of love to you. I will inspire you. But I cannot do the work for you. You yourself will have to do the work. The struggle and exertion must come from your side."

If one feels ready for a guru—that is, one is following the *yamas* and *niyamas* (yoga's ethical practices) and has gone as far as possible on the path of yoga without help—then one should sincerely pray for a guru and watch one's dreams. One should remember that the guru may not be convenient or may not look or act the way one expects. Until meeting the guru, one should continue learning from a qualified teacher and polishing one's conduct.

As Swami Rama wrote in his autobiography, "We should not worry about who will guide us. The question is: Am I prepared to be guided? Jesus had only 12 close disciples. He helped many, but he imparted the secret wisdom only to those few who were prepared. The Sermon on the Mount is comprehended by only a few, not by the multitudes. Those not on the path do not understand, for example, why one should be meek and poor.

"You'll never meet a bad guru if you are a good student. But the reverse is also true; if you are a bad student, you won't meet a good guru. Why should a good guru assume responsibility for a bad student? Nobody collects garbage. If you are in search of a guru, search within first. To become a yogi means to know your own condition here and now, to work with yourself. Don't grumble because you don't have a teacher. Ask whether you deserve one. Are you capable of attracting one?"

Make an Offering: Karma Yoga

"Service to others is the rent you pay for your room here on Earth."
—Muhammad Ali

Back in 2004, my asana practice at the Ashtanga Yoga Research Institute in Mysore, India, was focused on standing up from backbend. Sharath Jois, then assistant director of the institute, had told me that once I could do this consistently, I'd be able to practice Ashtanga's intermediate series.

So, every day I'd practice primary series and try to stand up from backbends. One day, when this was exceptionally difficult, I found myself repeatedly falling down and was about to give up. Then I looked over at the large images of Lord Ganesh and Lord Ram on the *shala* (studio) windows and silently addressed them: "This one is for you."

Next thing I knew I was standing up, as if propelled by an unseen force.

On another day in Mysore, I felt like I was getting sick and went to my pharmacist for some medication. He gave me some digestion medication and said it should work within 24 hours. It did, and when I went back to thank him, he gestured towards the sky and said, "I did nothing."

In other words, he was acting as an instrument of God—or the universe. Something similar had happened to me with backbends; on some level, I'd stopped struggling and let go of focusing on the outcome. I'd surrendered.

This is the path of *Karma* yoga, or selfless action, as outlined in the *Bhagavad-Gita*, which says, "To work, alone, you are entitled, never to its fruit. Neither let your motive be the fruit of action, nor let your attachment be to non-action." This means that we should perform our duties without attachment since the outcome is not in our hands. It is similar to the Christian idea of "Thy will be done," or aligning oneself with the universal or divine will.

Karma yoga is one of the four main paths of yoga and the easiest to follow for householders (lay persons) and those who are active in the world. It is said to be the quickest way to dissolve the ego or sense of separation, which is one of the things yogis believe keeps us from experiencing lasting peace and happiness. On a practical level, Karma yoga takes us out of our own heads and helps us see the common thread that binds everything together; it moves us from aloneness towards oneness.

In class, we can do this by offering our asana practice to something unselfish, such as dedicating it to someone who is suffering or to an ideal—or the highest practice of all: dedicating it to God or the Supreme Self (the spark of the divine that resides in every living being).

"If you practice any aspect of yoga for selfish reasons, it's not really yoga at all, according to the *Bhagavad-Gita*," my guru, Sri Dharma Mittra, said in a February 2017 interview with *Yoga Journal* magazine. "Anytime we are able to make our practice an offering, our practice becomes really powerful. Experiencing this leads to lots of enthusiasm to pursue and keep at it. The secret of success in yoga practice is constant practice. Success in practice will lead to inner peace, which will have a great effect on everything, eventually leading to peace for all, everywhere."

I once explained this concept to a group of yoga teacher trainees, and one of them jumped in with a personal example. A criminal defense attorney, he said that he practices a version of Karma yoga every day: he makes the best case he can before the judge and jury, and then must let go of the outcome, or verdict.

"The difference between regular action where there is always expectation and Karma Yoga is truly the mental attitude," Sri Dharma Mittra said.

As he explained in a 2012 interview, "When I first began doing Karma yoga, I had already heard that it had to be offered as a completely selfless action. In the beginning, even though it looks from the outside as though we renounce any physical benefits or rewards inherent in the actions we are supposedly offering to others, deep down inside we are always interested in spiritual rewards and there is always a 'little string' attached. As we grow and evolve spiritually, spend time near the Guru, gain more knowledge and are engaged in constant practice, we come to realize there should be no string at all. We expect nothing and hope to receive no spiritual benefits. With a little bit of Self-Knowledge and as we get a little bit closer to Self-realization, the ego disappears and automatically the Karma yoga becomes perfect and is performed without any expectation. We do everything because it has to be done for the sake of the Self, not expecting anything."

There's a wonderful story about oil magnate John D. Rockefeller meeting Swami Vivekananda in 1894. The swami said that the money Rockefeller had earned did not belong to him and suggested that he use it to do good in the world. Initially annoyed at the swami's brashness, Rockefeller returned a week later and showed him his plans to donate a large sum of money to a public institution—his first such effort—then waited for the swami to thank him. Instead, Swami Vivekananda said, "It is for you to thank me."

In other words, Karma yoga does not mean making grand gestures and boasting about them in your bio or doing good for a tax deduction or to secure a wing of a hospital in your name; rather, service is done for the sake of service. My spiritual mother used to tell a story about waiting for a flight at the airport with Sri Dharma when someone near them became ill and began to vomit. Sri Dharma was quick to offer help before anyone else acted.

If you are ever feeling sorry for yourself or have a strong sense of entitlement, volunteering or donating money or helping someone in need can quickly transform those feelings into gratitude. Karma yoga can also mean helping a spiritual teacher, fellow aspirant, or organization.

On a very basic level, Karma yoga means serving others anonymously in small ways, whenever possible, such as letting someone go ahead of you in traffic, giving up your seat to an older person, blessing someone when they sneeze, giving a compliment, or praying or doing your spiritual practice for others.

Any activity—including one's job—can be a form of Karma yoga. The important thing is to do it to the best of your ability and without attachment. (This does not mean you should stagnate in your work or not stand up for yourself or not ask for a raise or promotion when it is due; it means doing what is right and letting go of the results.)

Karma yoga has many benefits. Sri Dharma says it can be even better than meditation and is an essential step on the path towards liberation. "Acting in this way, one gradually loses all selfishness and notions such as: 'I am the doer,'" he explained in a 2010 New Year's message. "Thus comes total surrender of the ego. Why do selfless service? Because without it, there will be no union, absorption or Self-realization…."

In addition, according to the laws of karma and reincarnation, selfless action creates no new karma that must be paid back later. The *Bhagavad-Gita* says, "He who does actions, offering them to the Absolute and abandoning attachment, is free from error."

You may find that the more you give up doership of your actions (having the feeling that you are acting alone), the more the universe will start to work with you (rather than against you).

"There is nothing chaotic or capricious in this world," said Swami Sivananda. "Things do not happen in this universe by accident or chance in a disorderly manner. They happen in regular succession and events follow each other in a regular order. There is a kind of definite connection between what is being done now by you and what will happen in the future. Sow always the seeds which will bring pleasant fruits and which will make you happy herein and hereafter."

Additional Resources

The *Bhagavad-Gita* translated by Swami Nikhilananda
Karma Yoga by Swami Vivekananda
Practice of Karma Yoga by Swami Sivananda
How Can I Help? by Ram Dass
volunteermatch.org or idealist.org

Mantra and Japa

"The name of God, chanted correctly or incorrectly, knowingly or unknowingly, carefully or carelessly, is sure to give the desired result. The glory of the name cannot be established through reasoning and intellect. It can certainly be experienced or realized only through devotion, faith and constant repetition of the name. Every name is filled with countless potencies or shaktis [powers]."
—Swami Sivananda

There's an ancient story in yoga about a man who asked a *sadhu* (holy person) to give him a genie who could fulfill his every wish. The sadhu agreed, but told the man he must keep giving the genie things to do or the genie would eat him. When the genie appeared, the man asked him to build him a palace, which took only a few seconds. The man then asked for servants, food, and everything else he could think of. In a short time, the man ran out of desires and the genie was ready to eat him.

Panicking, the man called upon the sadhu for help. The sadhu pulled a curly hair from his head and told the genie to straighten it and stand it on end. The genie tried and tried without success. But he became completely absorbed in his task and left the man alone.

In this tale, the genie represents the mind when it is out of control, while the effort to straighten a curly hair is the practice of repeating *mantra*—a sacred word or set of syllables used in prayer or meditation.

Mantra, *bhajans* (hymns), and *kirtan* (call-and-response chanting) are part of the devotional or *bhakti* path of yoga. These practices are direct, easy, and suitable for everyone. In the ancient Sanskrit language, the meaning of a word is not considered to be separate from its sound, and each of the alphabet's 50 letters has a specific vibration that affects the body and mind.

"All mantras have the same power if done with the correct attention," says Sri Dharma Mittra in his book *Yoga Wisdom*. "The point," he writes, "is to rest the thoughts on God alone without interruption. This is realization."

Spiritual teacher and author Eknath Easwaran (1910–1999) called mantra (also known as *mantram*) "a powerful spiritual formula, which, when repeated silently in the mind, has the capacity to transform consciousness. There is nothing magical about this. It is simply a matter of practice. The mantram is a short, powerful spiritual formula for the highest power that we can conceive of—whether we call it God, or the ultimate reality, or the Self within. Whatever name we use, with the mantra we are calling up what is best and deepest in ourselves. The mantram has appeared in every spiritual tradition, West and East, because it fills a deep, universal need in the human heart."

Indeed, the *Bible* says, "Whosoever shall call upon the name of the Lord shall be saved" (Acts 2:21), while the *Quran* states, "Glorify the name of your Lord, the Most High" (87.1).

I was feeling a little despondent after returning from India in 2017. So, I decided to chant the "Mahishasura Mardini Stotram" in addition to my usual evening practices. Written by the 8th-century Indian saint Adi Shankaracharya, the vigorous Sanskrit hymn tells the story of the goddess Durga slaying a buffalo demon who represents our lower nature. When I finished the chant, I felt blissful and energized (and continued to chant it nearly nightly for several months).

But mantra need not be complicated or even uttered aloud. Easwaran, who experienced paralyzing stage fright before debate matches at college, asked his grandmother for advice. "She told me not to dwell on the anxiety, but just to keep repeating in my mind the words Rama, Rama, Rama," he wrote in his 1977 *Mantram Handbook*. "I wasn't a particularly devout young man, and my unspoken reaction to my granny's advice was, 'That's too easy, too simple, too miraculous.' I was skeptical, but such was my love for my grandmother that I tried it anyway." It worked, and Easwaran continued to chant it for the rest of his life.

Choosing a mantra

Choose a mantra you have an affinity for, use it regularly, and stick with it, since changing mantras diminishes their effect. It is also more effective to use an existing mantra that has a history and tradition, rather than making something up.

The simplest Sanskrit mantra is *Om*, or *Aum*. Most longer Sanskrit mantras begin and end with Om; it is considered to be the first and highest of all mantras, or divine words.

The word Om has four parts. The first is the "A," which sounds like the "a" in father and is pronounced in the throat with the mouth wide open; it is usually fairly short. The second is the "u," which rhymes with home and is pronounced with the mouth actively shaped like an "o." Then the mouth closes slowly and the sound becomes the "m," creating a pleasant vibration. The fourth is the silence that follows. Sri Dharma Mittra, says that during the silence one should focus on the vibration behind the forehead and that practicing this way for ten minutes or longer can reduce symptoms of depression (see "Om, the Sacred Pravana").

Om and all the mantras that spring from it are like asanas for the mouth and should be pronounced with care and concentration as well as with proper motivation and understanding. They should also be treated with respect, whether one believes in them or not.

There are Sanskrit mantras for every temperament and situation:

- "Om Gam Ganapataye Namaha" is for Lord Ganesh, the remover of obstacles.
- "Om Namo Narayanaya" is for inner peace and world peace and invokes Lord Vishnu, the preserver of the universe.
- "Om Namah Shivaya" means "I bow to Shiva," who is considered the Supreme reality, or consciousness, in which everything resides.
- "Om Sri Durgayei Namaha" addresses the goddess Durga, also known as the Divine Mother, who symbolizes the positive, feminine energy that is used against the negative forces of wickedness and evil.
- "Soham" means "I am That; That I am" and is suitable for anyone, especially atheists and those who have an intellectual bent.

- "Om Mani Padme Hum" is a Buddhist mantra that means "Hail to the jewel in the lotus."

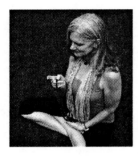

Japa on a mala

Japa, or the meditative repetition of a mantra or a divine name, can be done using a *mala,* a rosary that has 108 beads plus an extra one in the center called the "guru bead" (which is not counted). A mala can be used for general mantras like the ones above or for a personal mantra given to a *sadhaka* (seeker) by his or her spiritual preceptor. It can be repeated silently, whispered, or said aloud. While doing japa, I have had nausea, headaches, and fatigue—not to mention anxiety—disappear.

In my lineage, the mala, which should not touch the floor, is held in the right hand above the height of the navel. The index finger (which represents the ego) never touches the beads, which rest on the middle finger and are pulled toward oneself using the thumb. Start with a bead next to the guru bead and mentally repeat one mantra, then move the bead with the thumb, and repeat the mantra with the next bead. When you get to the end, you may continue by turning the mala at the guru bead and starting again with the bead you just counted. The left hand usually rests on the knee or lap in *jnana mudra* (index finger touching the thumb).

Whether you choose to mentally repeat a simple or complex mantra by yourself, or belt out a hymn with a group of people, it is bound to have an effect.

"Whenever you are angry or afraid, nervous or worried or resentful, repeat the mantram until the agitation subsides," wrote Easwaran. "The mantram works to steady the mind, and all these emotions are power running against you which the mantram can harness and put to work for you."

In his 2010 memoir, *Chants of a Lifetime,* Krishna Das wrote, "Once when I was on tour, somebody had stolen my laundry from the hotel washing machine. I was pissed. I had to leave for the kirtan without having found my favorite red T-shirt. But then I sat down and began to sing, and life immediately got very simple. All

I had to do was sing. It was very liberating. I didn't have to do anything else at the moment except sing and allow the Name to draw me within. How fantastic! And when I got back to the hotel, my laundry was back."

Finding Peace Through the Play of the Gunas

*"Again, the mind is in three states, one of which is darkness, called
Tamas, found in brutes and idiots; it only acts to injure. No other
idea comes into that state of mind. Then there is the active state of
mind, Rajas, whose chief motives are power and enjoyment. 'I will
be powerful and rule others.' Then there is the state called Sattva,
serenity, calmness, in which the waves cease, and the water of the
mind-lake becomes clear. It is not inactive, but rather intensely active.
It is the greatest manifestation of power to be calm."*
—Swami Vivekananda, *The Complete Works of Swami Vivekananda*

I once told a student I was giving an out-of-town workshop focused on relieving the winter blues. She wanted her Type A sister, who lives near the venue, to attend. But, she said, her sister suf-
fers from anxiety—not depression. "They're two sides of the same
coin," I tried to explain, as she looked at me blankly.

According *Samkhya* (one of the six systems of India philosophy), the universe consists of two realities: eternal spirit, or God
(*purusha*), and matter, or nature (*prakriti*). Everything in the material world is made up of prakriti.

Prakriti consists of three *gunas,* or qualities of nature. The
three gunas are *rajas* (passion or action), *tamas* (inertia), and *sattva* (harmony or peace). "Everything you can perceive or think is
the gunas," says my guru, Sri Dharma Mittra, in his 2017 book,
Yoga Wisdom. This includes emotions, places, food, weather, plan-
ets—all of it. "Even the subtlest gods are the gunas—the good
gunas!"

The gunas are always shifting and changing, although usually
one is prevailing at a given point in time. Emotion-wise, we may

feel depressed when tamas prevails. When rajas dominates, we may feel anxious.

Of course, rajas is necessary for movement and tamas is needed for rest. The mix is healthy when it's controlled by sattva. As Sri Dharma says, "Be established in sattva. It's a guna, but you have no choice—you're here in a body."

When tamas prevails, it is said to be like looking at the world through a paper bag; our perception is completely distorted. When rajas dominates, it is like looking through a wine bottle, a little clearer but still opaque and distorted. When sattva prevails, it's like looking through clear glass.

Tamas has been described in the *Bhagavad-Gita* as being like poison in the beginning and like poison in the end; it is painful or unpleasant from the outset as well as in the long run. It is the quality of selfish passivity and is associated with ignorance, laziness, stubbornness, depression, procrastination, greed, doubt, pessimism, and a lack of compassion; oversleeping and overeating are typical manifestations. Tamasic foods include those that hurt going down and hurt later on, as well as meat, eggs, fish, alcohol, onions, garlic, and overripe, canned, frozen, fermented, or stale food. Tamas is associated with the colors black, gray, and dark blue. One may say that a formerly bustling city such as Detroit is tamasic.

Rajas is described as being like nectar in the beginning and poison in the end; it is initially pleasant but ultimately causes pain. It is the quality of selfish action or passion, and is associated with anxiety and nervous energy, willfulness, and materialistic desires; by-products can include craving, attachment, and suffering. It is driven by the ego and is characterized by attachment to the fruits of one's actions; it is associated with heat, passion, enterprise, ambition, restlessness, and constant activity and movement. Rajasic foods are dry, sour, bitter, salty, and fried—foods that inflame the senses; they include salt, hot peppers, onions, garlic, chocolate, and coffee. Eating too quickly is also rajasic. Rajas is associated with the color red. New York City, "the city that never sleeps," may be considered rajasic.

Sattva is said to be like poison in the beginning and nectar in the end; the initial self-control that is required may be difficult, but the results are pleasant. Sattva is the quality of peace, calm, balance, purity, and harmony and is characterized by self-control, wisdom, benevolence, and a serene, detached mind. Sattvic foods are mild, fresh, nourishing, easily digested, and light and include fresh vegetables; cereals; sprouted nuts, grains, and beans; and ripe, juicy fruit. Sattva is associated with the color white. A calm and pleasant place such as an ashram or an outdoor natural setting may be considered sattvic.

Fortunately, the gunas can be managed when they adversely affect the body and emotions. In yoga, we use rajas to break through tamas, and we use sattva to balance rajas.

When I tapered off antidepressants over a decade ago, I used the pranayama, concentration, and meditation practices I learned from my guru to manage my moods. (I also quit while under the care and guidance of an MD and therapist, after doing a lot of research and concocting an elaborate plan for how I would deal with any fallout.) When I felt anxious, I did the grounding Ashtanga primary series and Sri Dharma's calming breathing. When I was lethargic and depressed, I did Ashtanga's invigorating intermediate series and Sri Dharma's positive breathing. When I felt balanced, I did Sri Dharma's more integrated asana practice and alternate nostril breathing.

It worked surprisingly well, and I never looked back.

Not long after I took that step, a yoga studio owner noticed the change in me and invited me to lead a workshop for people who suffer from anxiety and winter blues. I've been teaching—and refining—the workshop ever since.

Remember, the gunas are found in everything we perceive, including the sound *Aum,* or *Om.* In Om, the "A" is rajas (action), "u" is sattva (harmony), and "m" is tamas (inertia); the silence that follows is *turiya,* comparable to purusha, which is beyond these three states. Sri Dharma says, "What you really are is action-less, perception-less. You are moving according to your previous conditions; gunas acting with the gunas, but you are separate—the Witness."

Practice

To balance tamas, go to yoga class (do not stay home) and, if possible, find an active, energizing class that includes such things as sun salutations, *vinyasa* (flow), backbends, handstands, and/or spinal twists. At home, listen to active and uplifting music, and move to it. Wear bright colors, spend time in the sun, and avoid negative people. Try something new; visit an unfamiliar place, such as a café, museum, or neighborhood. Or chant Om for 10 minutes, while focusing on the third eye. (Learn more in "Weathering Winter Gracefully.")

To balance rajas, slow down. Listen to sattvic (calm) music. Breathe deeply through the nose. Wear light or pastel colors or white. Do a calm and grounding practice that includes forward bends, long holds, inversions, and a long *savasana* (relaxation). Avoid caffeine and stimulating environments. Walk (don't run) in nature.

To further cultivate sattva, adopt a mild, healthy, and fresh diet that consists primarily of fruit, vegetables, legumes, whole grains, and other natural foods. Sri Dharma says, "Food affects the gunas. Even your spiritual knowledge can be blocked [because of your diet]." (To learn more, see "Eat Like a Yogi.")

Most important, take time to meditate several times a day, even just for a moment. Be still and observe which guna is prevailing in your body and mind, without getting caught up in it. Do this knowing that it will change, and that the act of observation is more important than what you notice.

Eventually you may find that you start to identify with the inner witness and not with the play of the gunas. "When an individual overcomes the three gunas, he or she neither likes harmony, illumination, activity, or delusion when they are present, nor dislikes them when they are absent," says Sri Dharma Mittra. "He or she remains unshaken and unconcerned, knowing that the gunas are carrying out their actions. Alike in pleasure and pain, remaining the same towards a piece of gold or a lump of clay, towards the desirable and the undesirable, equal in defamation and self-adulation, alike in honor and dishonor, the same to friends and foes, without any egoistic effort in performing efforts."

The *Bhagavad-Gita* says, "When the embodied soul has risen above the three gunas of which its body is made, it gains deliverance from birth, death, old age, and pain and becomes immortal."

Nadis, Chakras, and the Subtle Body

"The chakras are the states of consciousness."
–Sri Dharma Mittra

I first heard about the *chakras* back in the 1980s. To me—a mohawk-sporting punk rocker—it sounded like a lot of hippie talk.

But many years later I heard about *nadis*, chakras, and the subtle body from my guru, Sri Dharma Mittra, and it suddenly made sense.

"The *nadis* are subtle conduits or channels through which the energy flows," Sri Dharma explained in his 2017 book, *Yoga Wisdom*. "They are also called psychic channels, and they are not visible to the physical eyes. The 72,000 nadis are like insulated wires or pipes with three layers. The main psychic channel is called *sushumna*, located in the spinal column, starting at the base of the spine and extending to the crown of the head. Its main purpose is to serve as a passage for the *kundalini* power [primal energy] in its journey to the *sahasrara* or crown chakra.

"There are two other important channels: *ida* and *pingala*, through which the solar and lunar energies flow. Ida is the white channel and pingala is the red. These channels run from the nostrils to the base of the spine, intersecting each other and also at sushumna which is between them at precise locations. These points of intersection are said to be the major chakras…The chakras really look like auras, each of a different color—not like the drawings with the petals. The major chakras are like flowers facing down until the *prana* [vital life force] passes through them, and then they bloom."

The chakras and nadis are part of the subtle, or astral, body, which is the same size and shape as the physical body but is not visible to the eye. (Yogis believe we have three bodies—the physical, subtle, and causal. The causal body is the most complex; it is like a computer hard drive that contains all of our deeds, karmas, tendencies, etc. from the past and transports the essence of the individual from one life into the next incarnation. It is from the causal body that the physical and astral bodies arise.) The subtle body's energy channels correspond to the nerves and blood vessels; some are said to be finer than 1/1000 of a hair. It is through these nadis that our consciousness manifests.

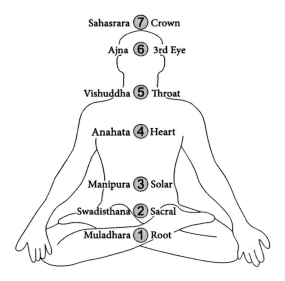

Sahasrara ⑦ Crown
Ajna ⑥ 3rd Eye
Vishuddha ⑤ Throat
Anahata ④ Heart
Manipura ③ Solar
Swadisthana ② Sacral
Muladhara ① Root

The nadis begin at *kanda* at the base of the spine; ida (which is the feminine, cooling, negative energy) ends at the left nostril, while pingala (the masculine, heating, positive energy) ends at the right. Prana moves through the nadis. Take a moment and check which of your nostrils is more open right now, left or right? In a healthy body, the open side switches off every couple of hours. Usually, we are more awake and alert when the right one is open, and more tired when the left is; that is why yogis like to have the right side open when they eat (to stoke the digestive fire) and the calming left side open when they go to sleep.

Yogis balance these two energies and encourage the prana, kundalini or *shakti* (latent) energy to move up the spine through *pranayama*, or breath control practices, which are learned from a guru or qualified teacher. To practice safely, one must first purify the mind and body.

"Aspirants must have all the *sattvic* [calm, pure] qualities and should be quite free from impurities," writes Swami Sivananda in his classic *Kundalini Yoga*. "*Satsanga* [holy company], seclusion, dietetic discipline, good manners, good character, *brahmacharya* [celibacy], *vairagya* [nonattachment], etc., form the strong foundation of yogic life. The help of a guru, who has already trodden the path, is absolutely necessary for quick progress on the spiritual path."

He continues, "Before awakening the kundalini, you must have *deha suddhi* (purity of body), nadi suddhi (purity of the nadis), *manas* suddhi (purity of mind), and *buddhi* suddhi (purity of the intellect)."

Sri Dharma stresses practicing *yama* (nonharming, truthfulness, nonstealing, continence, and nongreed) and *niyama* (internal and external purity, contentment, self-discipline, self-study, and surrender of the ego). Asana, pranayama, chanting, meditation, *mudras* (hand gestures), *bandhas* (internal locks), *Karma* yoga (selfless service), and *Bhakti* yoga (yoga of devotion) are also helpful for opening the nadis and balancing the chakras.

The nadis meet at intersections called chakras (wheels), or swirling vortexes of energy. The chakras are said to control the organs and glands located near them. Each chakra corresponds to a location, color, element, presiding deities, and *bija* (seed) *mantra* (one-syllable sound).

The energy moves up and down the chakras according to our past and current actions, traveling upward as the nadis are purified and our consciousness rises. Stress, unethical behavior, and other factors can lead to imbalances or stuck or downward-moving energy, as can poor diet, sedentary living, negative thinking, and strong emotions such as anger, hatred, greed, fear, and worry.

Sri Dharma says that when the energy is at the *muladhara* chakra (located at the base of the spine), we are interested in survival. When the energy is at the second chakra (three inches below

🪷	1 Muladhara Chakra	2 Swadhisthana Chakra	3 Manipura Chakra
Meaning	root	one's own seat	jewel city
Location	base of spine	sacrum (3" below navel)	solar plexus
Color	red (four-petal lotus)	orange (six-petal lotus)	yellow (ten-petal lotus)
Gland	adrenals (fight-or-flight response)	testes and ovaries	pancreas (blood sugar)
Primary Functions	survival, grounding, smell	creativity, sexual energy, desire, pleasure, stability, self-confidence, well-being, taste	will, determination, assertion, personal power, joy, anger, sight
Element	earth	water	fire
Presiding Deities	Lord Ganesh, Dakini	Lord Brahma, Rakini	Lord Vishnu, Lakini
Helpful Poses/ Practices	*pascimottanasana* (intense back stretch), *mula bandha* (root lock)	*balasana* (child's pose), *anjaneyasana* (monkey pose), *uddiyana bandha* (navel lock)	*navasana* (boat), *kapalabhati* (shining skull breathing)
Seed Mantra	*Lam*	*Vam*	*Ram*

4 Anahata Chakra	5 Vishuddha Chakra	6 Ajna Chakra	7 Sahasrara Chakra
unstruck	especially pure	command	thousand-petaled
center of chest (heart)	base of throat	between eyebrows, 3" behind forehead	crown of head
green (12-petal lotus)	blue (16-petal lotus)	indigo or violet (two petals)	violet or white (thousands of petals)
thymus (immune system)	thyroid (growth)	pineal (melatonin)	pituitary, hypothalamus
love, compassion, wisdom, touch, mental patience and equilibrium, wisdom	creativity, communication, expression, eloquence, synthesis, hearing	direct perception, intuition, imagination, visualization, concentration, self-mastery	union, bliss, sense of empathy/oneness, superconscious state
air	space	(mind)	(consciousness)
Isha/Rudra, Kakini	Sadashiva, Sakini	Paramashiva (Shambu), Hakini	Lord Shiva, Yakini
backbends	shoulderstand and fish	headstand (focus on third eye)	meditation
Yam	*Ham*	*Om*	none

the navel in the center of the spine) we are focused on sexual matters. At *manipura* (height of the navel), we are interested in name, fame, and power. At *anahatha* (heart center), we are compassionate. When it's at *vishuddha* (base of throat), we become serious about spiritual matters. When it's at the *ajna* chakra (third eye, between the eyebrows), we have divine perception. (Note: Forcing the kundalini to move up before one has achieved sufficient purity can result in debilitating, lifelong physical and mental problems.)

"Until you arrive at ajna chakra, you are always moving between them," he says.

Meditation is key to the process of moving energy through the chakras. "Through systematic meditation one can awaken the third eye and touch the cosmic awareness," writes Amit Ray in *Meditation: Insights and Inspirations*. "Sushumna nadi is the subtle pathway in the spinal cord which passes through the main psychic centers. The awakening of these centers means a gradual expansion of awareness, until it reaches the cosmic awareness. Each center has its own beauty and gracefulness. Through generations of ignorance and unconsciousness, this channel of awareness becomes obscured and hidden. Meditation is to become aware about this internal life energy. Meditation is the procedure to rearrange, harmonize, activate, and integrate the individual life energy with the cosmic life energy."

Part Five: Diet, Health, and Healing

Change Your Breathing, Change Your Life

"When the breath wanders the mind also is unsteady. But when the breath is calmed the mind too will be still, and the yogi achieves long life. Therefore, one should learn to control the breath."
—The *Hatha Yoga Pradipika*

When I waitressed at a vegetarian restaurant back in the early '90s, we got to know our regulars well. One day Gary, who always sat alone at booth six, seemed a lot more outgoing and energetic than usual; he also appeared to be glowing with peace and happiness. The staff noticed the change right away, and we figured he'd finally found a romantic partner. His answer surprised us.

"I learned to breathe," he said, beaming at us. "It's changed my life."

We just stared at him, uncomprehending. It didn't make sense to me then—this was a few years before I walked into my first yoga class—but now it does.

Yogis have long known that deep, full diaphragmatic (belly) breathing is the key to calming the mind and maximizing the function of every system of the body. It can also improve brain function, aid digestion and sleep, increase energy, reduce anxiety, lower blood pressure, improve posture, reduce food cravings, and help slow the aging process.

Yet, many of us breathe shallowly, either using the upper front lobes of the lungs rather than the diaphragm, doing thoracic (chest) breathing using the intercostal muscles, or doing clavicular breathing using the shoulders and collarbones. This inferior, shallower breathing can lead to increased stress; high blood pressure; and poor posture, digestion, and brain function, sapping our energy and taking a toll on every system of the body.

In Gopala Krishna's book *The Yogi: Portraits of Swami Vishnu-devananda*, Swami Vishnu drives this point home. One day the swami went to see a young Muhammad Ali sparring at a gym in Florida.

"His sparring partner took many punches, very strong punches," said Swami Vishnu. "Ali kept giving them one after another. Occasionally he would lean against the rope. Why? He was resting. Because his breathing was very shallow, he wasn't able to get sufficient oxygen and a few of his powerful punches took tremendous energy.

"After the fighting, I gave him an autographed copy of my book and said to him, 'You know, your breathing is very shallow. You won't be able to fight long if you don't change your breathing pattern.' I advised him in a friendly way, teaching him how to breathe and telling him, 'Increase your breathing capacity if you want to survive.'"

Deep and conscious belly breathing is the most basic form of *pranayama*, the fourth limb of the Ashtanga yoga or eight-limb system of *Raja* yoga (the royal path of yoga outlined in the *Yoga Sutras* of Patanjali). Yogis believe that the breath contains *prana*, or the vital life force. *Yama* means control; the practice of pranayama or control of this life force is one of the foundations of yoga in that it improves health and makes the mind calm and clear and prepares it for meditation.

Deep belly breathing makes full use of the diaphragm (the large, thin muscle that lies between the chest and belly and is considered the major muscle of breathing). When the diaphragm contracts, the lungs move downward, expand, and fill with air—pulling in prana. When the diaphragm relaxes and moves upward into the chest cavity and the intercostal muscles relax, space is reduced in the chest cavity, which forces carbon dioxide—rich air out of the lungs. We all breathed this way when we were babies and small children, before our chest muscles matured.

Ideally, this breathing is done through the nose, which filters, cleans, and humidifies the air before it enters the lungs. (Breathing through the nose can also improve digestion and reduce insomnia.)

Are you breathing consciously or unconsciously as you read this? The average person takes 15 breaths per minute, while some yogis take only a few breaths per minute.

Yogis believe that each person is assigned a certain number of breaths when they are born, according to their deeds from the past. When these breaths are used up, one's time is over. Therefore, breathing slowly means a longer life.

Indeed, the first thing we do when we're born is inhale; the last thing we do upon expiring is exhale. One of the few things we can control in between is the breath. In fact, breathing is the only physiological process that is both voluntary (you can control it) and involuntary (it will take care of itself if you don't).

"The body can't operate without the breath, so if conscious control of the breath is abandoned, then some unconscious part of the mind reflexively begins to function and starts breathing for us," wrote Swami Rama and physicians Rudolph Ballentine and Alan Hymes in the 1979 classic *Science of Breath: A Practical Guide.* "In this case, breathing falls back under control of the primitive parts of the brain, an unconscious realm of the mind where emotions, thoughts, and feelings, of which we may have little or no awareness, become involved and can wreak havoc with the rhythm of the breath. The breath may become haphazard and irregular when we lose conscious control of it."

By the same token, we can calm and even diffuse strong emotions by breathing deeply for several minutes—and feel a little bit "high," like Gary from the restaurant. "Feelings come and go like clouds in a windy sky. Conscious breathing is my anchor," wrote Thich Nhat Hanh in *Stepping into Freedom: An Introduction to Buddhist Monastic Training.*

Diaphragmatic breathing also has a powerful effect on the body, improving oxygenation of and blood flow to every system. It reduces tension and tightness in the neck and shoulders, and because those muscles are able to relax, it improves posture. It massages the internal organs, which improves digestion and drainage of lymph. Deep breathing also increases the secretion of growth hormone, which may slow the aging process. It helps lower blood pressure and blood sugar and improves mental function by increasing blood flow to the prefrontal cortex of the brain. It's also believed to reduce the stress hormones cortisol and adrenaline and improve the quality of sleep.

If that's not enough to convince you, when my guru, Sri Dharma Mittra, was asked at the 2009 Yoga Journal conference about how to stop overeating, he responded, "Do calm breathing (a simple deep breathing practice) and sing to the Lord."

Fortunately, it's easy to relearn how to breathe consciously.

Practice

There are many types of pranayama; most, like these, are done through the nose (with the mouth closed). The two listed below are safe, simple, and suitable for just about everyone.

Diaphragmatic breathing: To relearn how to breathe deeply, lie on your back as in *savasana* (corpse pose), with your hands on the belly and the tips of the middle fingers meeting just above the navel. Close the eyes and exhale through the nose. Now, begin breathing deeply (through the nose) into the belly. When you inhale, the fingers will separate and the rib cage will expand out to the sides. When you exhale, the navel will sink downward and the fingers will move back together. Continue to breathe into the belly for five to ten minutes or longer.

Make it a habit. Set your phone or computer's alarm clock to sound several times a day, at regular intervals. Each time you hear the alarm, breathe consciously into the belly for a minute or two (do not hit the snooze button!). After a few weeks, you will begin to do this automatically—and will have retrained your body how to breathe properly.

Three-part or complete breathing: Three-part breathing brings awareness to the three lobes of the lungs: upper, middle, and lower (we focus on the lower lobe in diaphragmatic breathing). To practice, lie down in savasana with the arms resting alongside the body (or, place the left hand on the belly and the right hand on the chest). Exhale completely. Inhale deeply into the belly. First, fill the abdomen (lower lobe), then the ribcage (middle lobe), and, finally, fill the chest and lift it toward the chin (upper lobe). As you exhale, reverse the order: empty the chest, allow the rib cage to contract, and let the navel sink toward the earth. Repeat 12 times.

Five Reasons to Eat Less Meat

*"Nonviolence leads to the highest ethics, which is the goal
of all evolution. Until we stop harming all other
living beings, we are still savages."*
—Thomas A. Edison

Becoming a vegetarian is a personal choice that more and more Americans are making; between 25 and 30 percent of Americans are now vegetarian, vegetarian-leaning, or vegetarian-inclined.

I gave up meat back in 1987—ten years before walking into my first yoga class. I grew up on a farm and got to know pigs, cows, sheep, goats, and other animals as individuals with unique personalities. We showed our pigs at the county fair, and when we learned that our prize-winning barrows had been auctioned off to become the centerpiece of a company barbeque, my stepbrother and I hugged our pigs and cried. (Then we went home and ate our usual diet of Oscar Mayer meat and fresh fish caught in our lake.)

A decade later, I spent a semester in Madrid and attended the bullfights every week. One Sunday my friend and I spied on what happened to the once-majestic bulls after the fight in a nondescript shack behind the bullring. Peering through a hole in the wall, we saw them hung from hooks, skinned, and unceremoniously butchered into innocuous-looking cuts of meat. The reality of it sunk in slowly, and two years later, I gave up eating beef and other mammals.

That summer, during a visit to Minneapolis in sweltering heat, I found myself stuck in traffic next to a truck full of live chickens; the stench was horrible. But that was nothing compared to what we saw and heard; the chickens sticking their heads out of their overcrowded cages, gasping for air. I immediately saw the connection between my diet and their sad fate, and gave up poultry that very day. I quit eating fish a few months later, after being offered a platter of fresh paella in Madrid, with the eyes still on the prawns staring at me. I quit eating eggs in 2007, during my first teacher training with Sri Dharma Mittra—who said they contain the same material as chicken ("they're embryos").

I stopped eating animals gradually, which worked well for my temperament (I don't like sudden change). I did it out of compassion for the animals, and because I saw my role in their suffering. But there are many reasons to consider giving up eating meat either on a full-time or a part-time basis, either gradually or all at once, according to your circumstances and temperament. Here are just a few of them:

1. Compassion

Ahimsa or nonharming of living beings is the first part of the first step, the *yamas*, of the eight limbs of yoga. (The yamas, or ethical roots of yoga, are to be practiced in word, thought, and deed, regardless of time, place, or circumstance.) The Buddha said that all beings love life and tremble in fear at violence. My guru, Sri Dharma Mittra, says that even if you don't actually kill the animal or bird or fish yourself, if you eat it you are participating in this violence. He also says that all of the other virtues stem from compassion; indeed, one of the highest yoga practices is to put yourself in the place of others. (If you have trouble with this, view the animals up close at a farm or petting zoo. If that doesn't work, visit a slaughterhouse, as I did; you can do it either in person or online at websites such as www.peta.org.) Or consider that the U.S. Department of Agriculture estimates that in 2011, 9.1 billion cows, chickens, turkeys, ducks, pigs, and sheep were slaughtered for food. According to The Humane Society of the United States, about 1.4 billion animals could be spared each year if every American cut out meat just once a week.

2. To accelerate your spiritual practice

Yogis believe that the spark of the divine that is in each of us is also in every other living thing—including animals. This *atman*, or soul, is the same in everyone, whether they're a saint, a dog, or a criminal. Yogis believe that when we eat animals or hurt others, we are only hurting ourselves on a karmic level (we will pay later) and also because we are harming our own highest Self. When we do this, even though we know better, the spark of the divine shines a little less brightly in us.

3. For peace of mind

Eating meat can make it difficult to meditate. My guru has noted that animals experience fear and anger when they are slaughtered, and that when we eat meat we ingest those same emotions. He says it makes Self-realization all but impossible. "If you eat animals too much, you cannot meditate. The mind is in a cave, in darkness. You do not feel the vibration or the presence of God because you are blocking your psychic channels and senses of perception, which are very subtle. It prevents the bliss from coming out."

4. For the health of the planet

The U.N.'s Food and Agriculture Organization and other organizations have determined that factory farming has made animal agriculture the number one contributor to global warming—more so than all of the world's cars, trains, and planes combined. Production of meat is "one of the top two or three causes of all of the most serious environmental problems, both global and local: air and water pollution, deforestation, loss of biodiversity," wrote Jonathan Safran Foer in a 2009 *New York Times Magazine* article, "Against Meat." "Eating factory-farmed animals—which is to say virtually every piece of meat sold in supermarkets and prepared in restaurants—is almost certainly the single worst thing that humans do to the environment." Meat-eating has other long-term effects on the environment: "Around 30 percent of global biodiversity loss can be attributed to livestock production, such as the spread of pasture land or turning over forests and savannahs... to feed production," says Duncan Williamson, corporate stewardship manager at the World Wildlife Fund U.K. According to the PB&J Campaign, whose mission is to combat environmental destruction by reducing the amount of animal products people consume, eating a plant-based meal for lunch instead of a burger prevents 2.5 pounds of carbon dioxide emissions, saves 133 gallons of water, and preserves 24 square feet of land. According to the Environmental Defense Fund, "If every American had one meat-free meal per week, it would be the same as taking more than 5 million cars off our roads."

5. For your own health

A vegetarian diet can lower the occurrence of cancer, heart disease, diabetes, hypertension, osteoporosis, kidney stones, gallstones, and a litany of other diseases, according to the Physicians Committee for Responsible Medicine (PCRM). "Fatty red meats and many processed meats are high in saturated fat, which raises LDL (bad) cholesterol and increases the risk of coronary heart disease," says Rachel K. Johnson, a spokesperson for the American Heart Association and professor of Nutrition and Medicine at the University of Vermont. Based on a 20-year study, Caldwell Esselstyn Jr., M.D., described how eating a plant-based, oil-free diet can reverse the effects of heart disease in his 2007 book *Prevent and Reverse Heart Disease*. A study of 35,000 women published in the *British Journal of Cancer* found that those who ate the most red and processed meat had the highest risk of breast cancer, while other studies have linked meat consumption to colon, prostate, pancreatic, and gastric cancers. For more info, visit pcrm.org.

The protein myth

Concerned you won't get enough protein on a vegan or vegetarian diet? PCRM says that most Americans consume about double the protein their bodies need. "To consume a diet that contains enough, but not too much, protein, simply replace animal products with grains, vegetables, legumes (peas, beans, and lentils), and fruits. As long as one is eating a variety of plant foods in sufficient quantity to maintain one's weight, the body gets plenty of protein." For more info (and tasty, meat-free, high-protein recipes), visit pcrm.org.

Resources

There are myriad resources available for those considering a vegetarian diet. The Meatless Mondays website, meatlessmonday.com, has recipes and other resources. One of my favorite pages is called "How to Became a Vegetarian, the Easy Way" (zenhabits.net/how-to-become-a-vegetarian-the-easy-way/).

Other helpful sites include vegsource.com (Vegsource Interactive), vegsoc.org (UK Vegetarian Society), goveg.com (PETA), ivu.org (International Vegetarian Union), and vega-noutreach.org (Vegan Outreach). Many cities also have local vegetarian meet-up groups.

Helpful cookbooks include *The Yoga Cookbook: Vegetarian Food for Body and Mind* by the Sivananda Yoga Vedanta Centers, *How to Cook Everything Vegetarian* by Mark Bittman, *Vegetarian Supercook* by Rose Elliott, *Moosewood Restaurant Cooks at Home: Fast and Easy Recipes for Any Day* by the Moosewood Collective, and *Being Vegetarian for Dummies* by Suzanne Havala.

Eat Like a Yogi

"By the purity of food one becomes purified in his nature;
by the purification of his nature he verily gets memory
of the Self, and by the attainment of the memory of the Self,
all ties and attachments are severed."
—*Chandogya Upanishad*

Yogis have always believed that you are what you eat—literally. That's because the sheath that represents the physical body in yoga, called *anamaya kosha*, means the sheath made of food; it becomes, by extension, the mind. And only a *sattvic* (pure, calm) mind can help us fulfill our potential.

The *Gheranda Samhita* says, "Without observing moderation of diet, if one takes to the yogic practices, he cannot obtain any benefit but gets various diseases."

The *Bhagavad-Gita* says, "Yoga is not for him who eats too much nor for him who eats too little."

The *mitahara,* or moderate diet, means food should be simple and eaten in small quantities. At meals, the stomach's contents should consist of 50 percent food, 25 percent air, and 25 percent water. For better digestion, yoga's sister science, ayurveda, counsels us to avoid drinking liquid with meals (better to drink some warm water *after* eating) and to avoid cold drinks in general, as they impede digestion.

Traditionally, the best foods for yoga, meditation, and good health are *sattvic*: mild, substantial, fresh, pure, simple, and vegetarian. Sattvic foods include green vegetables, soaked nuts, fresh juices, whole grains, beans, root vegetables, leafy vegetables, and plenty of "good" oil, such as raw cold-pressed extra virgin olive oil, sesame oil, coconut oil, and flax seed oil. (For optimum absorption, fruit should be eaten alone and on an empty stomach.)

It can be difficult to maintain the self-control needed to keep a sattvic diet when tastier, less healthy, and more convenient options are available. In fact, one of the definitions of *sattva* is that it can be unpleasant in the beginning and yet become like nectar in the end (because it makes you feel good). I found this out firsthand a few years ago when my dinner hosts offered me a large slice of special cheesecake. Even though I wanted the whole slice, I ate only a tiny sliver, savoring each bit. The next morning I felt fine, while the other diners were bleary-eyed and crabby, complaining that consuming large quantities of the sugary delicacy kept them up most of the night.

The yogi tries to avoid stale, tasteless, putrid, rotten, and impure food, which is considered *tamasic,* (having the quality of inertia) and lacking in nutritional value.

Tamasic foods can include frozen, leftover, canned, processed, and twice-cooked foods as well as fast food, fried food, overly sweet food, and drugs and alcohol. These items are said to deplete the *prana* (life force). (I always knew this but continued to reheat food until I substantially cleaned up my diet—a process that took nearly three decades. One day after eating some reheated kitchari [moong dal and rice], I got in the car to drive somewhere and, even though I was well rested, nearly fell asleep at the wheel! After that, I largely avoided twice-cooked foods—and have had more energy ever since.)

Fish, eggs, meat, and foods that are bitter, sour, saline, or excessively hot, pungent, dry, or burning as well as coffee and tea, heavy spices, hot peppers, garlic, and onions are considered *rajasic* (having the quality of passion) and are thought to produce anger, passion, pain, and grief. They are also said to disturb the mind. (None of these foods are inherently bad—it's just that their consumption can have an undesirable effect on one's yoga practice and mental state.)

One of the definitions of *rajas* is that it can be pleasant in the beginning but becomes unpleasant in the end. This point was driven home on my first Belize retreat when we stopped in town after an excursion to Mayan ruins. One of the students came back to the van with an armful of chocolate and salty chips, which he shared with the others. About half an hour later, one of the students said he felt sick, adding "I think I get what you said now, about certain foods being nectar in the beginning and poison in the end."

To kindle the digestive fire and cleanse the stomach, try to begin each day with a drink of hot water and lemon, which may be sweetened with agave or maple syrup. Afterwards, you may have whatever you like. But you may find you no longer crave your usual caffeinated beverage.

Eating between meals should be minimized, as should eating heavy food after 6 p.m., which impedes digestion and makes the body feel heavy and stiff in the morning. A yogi also tries to avoid refined sugar; among other things, it makes the joints stiff. The largest meal is best enjoyed in the middle of the day. Kitchari is a tasty, nutritious, and easy-to-digest meal (see "Kitchari, Yoga's Wonder Food").

Meat is avoided because it is difficult to digest, it violates the tenet of *ahimsa* (nonharming of any living being in word, thought, or deed) and because one ingests the fear and anger the animal experienced at the time of death, which can disturb the mind.

Whenever possible, eat at regular times, at a moderate pace, and in a calm environment. Eating when hurried, angry, or upset adversely affects digestion. Try to chew each morsel of food 25 times before swallowing, especially if you have digestive issues or a tendency towards constipation.

If you do fall off your diet, don't beat yourself up. Just try to eat more cleanly the following day.

I have found that it is best to make changes to the diet slowly, because the mind and senses tend to rebel against a lot of sudden change.

Instead, try one or two of the things that are compatible with your temperament and lifestyle, and observe the effect after a few weeks. As with the rest of the ancient science of yoga, these practices should be applied and tested by each individual. Just be patient.

As Dharma Mittra says, "Move slowly, gently."

Resources
The Ayurvedic Cookbook by Amadea Morningstar

The Yoga Cookbook: Vegetarian Food for Body and Mind
    by Sivananda Yoga Vedanta Centers
*The Higher Taste: A Guide to Gourmet Vegetarian Cooking
    and a Karma-Free Diet* by ISKCON
The Hare Krishna Book of Vegetarian Cooking by Adiraja Dasa
The Path of Practice: A Woman's Book of Ayurvedic Healing
    by Bri Maya Tiwari

Kitchari, Yoga's Wonder Food

"Eat moderately what you know by experience is agreeable to you and what is digestible. Simple diet is best."
—Swami Sivananda

One of the best ways to detox, lose weight, and restore healthy digestion is by eating *kitchar*i (pronounced "kich-ah-ree"), a hearty, one-pot vegetarian stew of moong dal (split moong beans) and basmati rice.

This ancient, high-protein dish heals and soothes the digestive system, removes toxins, cleanses the blood and liver, and balances the metabolism. It may also assist in healthy weight loss. Plus it's a comfort food!

Kitchari (also spelled *khichadi* or *khichdi* or *khichri*) is a favorite of yogis (some believe its mild, healing qualities aid spiritual progress) and is also used in ayurvedic cleanses. It's commonly recommended for restoring health when one feels ill or is recovering from an illness and to end fasts. In addition, it balances all three *doshas*, or body types (*vata*, *pitta*, and *kapha*).

I started eating kitchari after ending up in the emergency room with blocked digestion in 2011; afterward I called my mentor, Chandra Om, founder of the Shanti Niketan Ashram and author of *The Divine Art of Nature Cure*. She made some suggestions that immediately restored me to health; one of them was to make kitchari a staple of my diet.

Since then I've eaten kitchari nearly every day, year-round—and it has healed my digestion. I alternate having it with brown basmati rice one day and white basmati rice the next. White rice is more healing and easier to digest, while brown is more nourishing; in addition, white rice is more cooling, while brown is more warming. I often bring kitchari with me in a Thermos when I'm out working all day, and when I travel I take a rice cooker that can be used to prepare it in a hotel room.

There are as many ways to make kitchari as there are to spell it. Although kitchari can be made with any legume, moong dal is the only legume that balances vata, or the quality of air/wind (in other words, it does not produce gas). Moong dal can be found online and at Indian grocery stores.

The first recipe below is based on how I make it for the purpose of healing the digestive tract. Feel free to experiment and season it the way you like. But keep in mind that adding too many ingredients will make it more difficult to digest.

Simple healing kitchari

Ingredients (serves one):
1/4 cup moong dal
1/3 cup uncooked brown basmati rice
    (or 1/4 cup uncooked white basmati)
1 tbsp cumin seeds
1 tbsp turmeric powder
2 tbsp ghee (clarified butter) or olive oil
3 cups water

Before cooking, sift through the rice and dal to remove any stones. Rinse each separately with at least 2 changes of water (rinse the white rice until the water is clear). Soak the rice and dal in water separately for at least two hours to remove air and gas.

Preparation with brown rice:
Heat 1 tbsp oil (or ghee) in pan. Add cumin seeds and heat until seeds begin to pop.

Add water, turmeric powder, rice, and dal. Heat to boiling. Cover and simmer for 40 minutes. Drain excess water. Add remaining oil and mix.

With white rice:
Follow the above instructions, but after cooking the cumin seeds, add the moong dal, turmeric powder, and water and cook for 20 minutes. Then add the white rice and cook for another 20 minutes.

You may also season your kitchari with ginger, coconut, fennel, or rosemary, or add vegetables like carrots, celery, or green beans. Just try to keep it simple (only a couple of extra ingredients).

Crock-Pot kitchari
To make it in a slow cooker, add the ingredients. Stir, cover, and cook on low for five hours.

Sivananda kitchari
(reprinted with permission from www.sivananda.org)

Ingredients (serves four):
1 cup moong dal
1 cup basmati rice
1 small piece ginger root
2 tbsp coconut shreds
1 bunch cilantro
6½ cups water
3 tbsp ghee
1 cinnamon stick
5 whole cardamom pods
5 whole cloves
10 whole black peppercorns
3 whole bay leaves
1/4 tsp turmeric powder
1/4 tsp salt

Wash dal and rice until water is clear. In a blender, put ginger, coconut, cilantro, and 1/2 cup of water and blend till liquefied.

Heat saucepan on medium heat. Add ghee, cinnamon, cardamom, cloves, peppercorns, and bay leaves. Stir for a moment, add blended

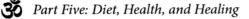

ingredients to spices, then add turmeric and salt. Stir until lightly browned.

Stir in moong dal and rice and mix well, add 6 cups of water, cover, bring to a boil. Let boil for 5 minutes. Then turn heat down to low and cook, lightly covered, until dal and rice are soft (25–30 minutes).

Additional resources
Ayurvedic Cooking for Self-Healing by Dr. Vasant Lad
The Yoga Cookbook by the Sivananda Yoga Vedanta Centers
The Ayurvedic Cookbook by Amadea Morningstar

Help for Insomnia

"When the world is itself draped in the mantle of night, the mirror of the mind is like the sky in which thoughts twinkle like stars."
—Khushwant Singh, *Delhi*

My first night in India was difficult. It took us 20 hours to get to Bangalore, and we were dazed when we arrived in the wee morning hours, only to find that our luggage was missing. After nearly two hours of pushing, shoving, and waiting, we finally filled out the necessary forms, met our friends, and checked in to a hotel, where I spent most of the night tossing and turning and didn't sleep a wink. My mind was reeling with worry and self-recrimination, and I wanted to go home. But then I started breathing deeply and imagining I was practicing Ashtanga yoga's primary series—and fell asleep before finishing the standing poses.

We've all experienced similar bouts of insomnia. Here are some tricks that have helped me over the years.

Practice

Regular yoga practice keeps the body in good working order, which makes just about everything in life easier, including sleep. Specific poses can also help. My guru, Sri Dharma Mittra, says that doing cobra pose and *dhanurasana* (bow) helps fight insomnia.

Viparita karani (legs-up-the-wall pose) prepares the body for sleep, and can be done right before bed—even on your bed if it's against a wall—for at least five minutes. If you're still not tired, follow it up with a short *savasana* (corpse pose) and/or *pranayama* (yogic breathing) and meditation. Child's pose and other supported forward bends can also have a calming effect.

Calming breathing, a type of *pranayama* recommended by my guru, slows down both body and mind. To perform it, sit up tall in a meditative posture with a straight spine. Empty the lungs completely. Then, inhale through both nostrils for a count of eight. Hold the breath for a count of four. Exhale through the nose for a count of eight. Continue for at least five minutes. (If the eight-four-eight count is difficult, inhale for a count of six, hold the breath for three counts, and exhale for six—or eliminate the breath holding.)

Another helpful practice: Concentrate on a candle flame before turning in. Place the flame at eye level, three feet away. Gaze at it and study it and fix it in your mind. Then close the eyes and continue to visualize the flame. Hold the image in your mind. When you lose the image, open the eyes, recapture it, and close them again, reproducing the image in your mind. Continue for several minutes.

My favorite sleep-inducing meditation is to count back from 30 (which can be done in bed if you wake up in the middle of the night). Visualize each number in any font or color or design that pleases you. If you lose count or get to zero, start again at 30. Continue until you feel sleepy or fall asleep.

Learn a *mantra* (word or phrase that's repeated) and say it to yourself when you cannot sleep or as part of your before-bed meditation. Swami Vishnudevananda recommended repeating "Om Namo Narayanaya" for world peace and inner peace. You can either imagine you are sending the mantra out to the world at large or that it's comforting you like a warm blanket (learn more in "Mantra and Japa").

Diet

Going to bed immediately after eating a high-protein meal may cause you to thrash about all night, as can drinking caffeinated beverages after 3 p.m. In the days when I ate garlic, it would keep me up all night, thirsty and irritable.

My guru says to avoid eating heavy food after 6 p.m. Try to stop eating, period, after 8 p.m. Otherwise the body will be busy digesting food when it should be resting.

A completely empty stomach can also keep you up at night. If you are hungry at bedtime, have a glass of warm milk. To make it even more effective stir in half a teaspoon of ginger powder, half a teaspoon of turmeric powder, and a quarter teaspoon of nutmeg. This traditional ayurvedic remedy induces sleep. Vegans may try eating a banana or drinking sour cherry juice; I have also had good results with Deglet Nour (or Noor) dates.

Applying raw sesame oil to the soles of the feet before bed is a time-tested *vata* (wind)-reducing cure for insomnia. Cover with a light pair of socks, so you don't make a mess.

Lifestyle

Clear out everything under your bed. "Anything in your energy field affects the quality of your sleep, so resist the temptation to stash junk under your bed," writes Karen Kingston in her 1999 book, *Clear Your Clutter with Feng Shui.* "If you have one of those beds that has drawers in it, the best thing you can keep in there is clean bed linen, towels or clothing."

Try to get up and go to bed at the same time each day. This includes eating at the same times each day. Being on a schedule worked when we were babies, and it remains effective at any age. (If you can't maintain a regular schedule and you have frequent insomnia, go to bed one hour later than usual.)

If what's keeping you up is noise, use earplugs, get a sleep sound machine, or put a white noise app on your phone (I also like to wear an eyeshade when I travel). Just make sure you set your alarm clock to go off at full volume. (That said, sleeping with an open window can help.)

If there is someone you have wronged or need to forgive, do so immediately; you'll sleep more soundly (learn more about forgiving in "Internal Spring Cleaning"). Following the *yama* (restraint) of *satya* (truthfulness), which includes things such as not lying on one's taxes, also makes it easier to sleep at night.

Take a warm bath before bed. Add a few teaspoons of raw sesame oil to soothe the skin.

Watch what you give your mind to play with just before bed. Avoid reading or watching material that is disturbing, thrilling, or frightening. It's far better to read or view something uplifting or inspiring just before nodding off.

Don't start a texting session right before bed, and make sure the phone is off when you retire.

During insomnia

Lie on your right side. This opens the left nostril and activates the *ida nadi* (left energy pathway), which is associated with the calming, cooling energy that helps induce sleep.

Try to avoid the urge to eat; it'll only keep you up longer. Avoid checking your phone.

Keep a pen and paper next to the bed and write down what is bothering you. Or copy down scripture. Breathe into your belly. Make the exhale twice as long as the inhale.

Try tricking your mind using paradoxical intention: instead of worrying about insomnia, focus on staying awake as long as you can.

Get some Mayan worry dolls. These tiny handcrafted dolls come in a small container that can be kept next to the bed. When you wake up, take them out and tell a worry or fear to each one. Then put them away. According to legend, they will worry about your problems while you sleep, and when you awaken, the problems will have been solved.

The C Word: Constipation

*"He who is temperate in his habits of eating, sleeping,
working and recreation can mitigate all material pains
by practicing the yoga system."*
—The *Bhagavad-Gita*

I've had trouble with digestion since I was a child. I remember staying with my grandmother and having my fecal matter compared with that of my best friend. Her healthy output got the thumbs-up, while my grandmother shook her head at my sad little "marbles." Then she gave me a tablespoonful of foul-tasting cod liver oil to lubricate my digestive system.

It probably didn't help that my first food was baby formula, which was soon replaced by the convenience foods that were the envy of my friends—instant breakfast, Space Food sticks, and frozen TV dinners. Although things improved as I cleaned up my diet over the years, it wasn't until my digestive system went on strike and I wound up in the emergency room some years ago that I really learned how to control constipation. Much of what helped came from my teacher and mentor, Chandra Om. Some of the techniques below are from her, as well as from naturopathy ("nature cure"), *ayurveda*, other teachers, and my own experience.

Yoga practices

Deep breathing into the belly is one of the easiest and most direct ways to improve overall digestion. Many of us breathe shallowly, using the upper, front part of the lungs. To relearn how to breathe properly, lie on your back with your hands on the belly and the middle fingers touching just above the navel. When you inhale into the belly, the middle fingers should separate. When you exhale, they should come back together. To train yourself to do this in daily life, set the alarm on your phone to go off several times during the day. Breathe deeply into the belly each time it goes off.

I learned sleeping baby pose from my preceptor, Sri Dharma Mittra. It is practiced right after eating, and is especially helpful for indigestion. To practice, lie on the belly, with the head turned to the right and the left hand turned up alongside the left hip. Frame the head with the right arm, and bend the right knee 90 degrees. This position places pressure on the stomach, which is on the left side of the abdomen. Stay in the pose for at least five minutes after eating (20 minutes is better).

A deep squatting pose such as *malasana* (garland pose) can have a laxative effect on the colon. To practice, stand and place the feet nearly mat-distance apart, toes turned out to the side. Squat down until the buttocks are a few inches from the floor (if this is difficult, stay up higher, place the buttocks on a block, or place a rolled blanket under the heels). Hold for five to 20 breaths. For better results, bring the feet parallel and rock back and forth.

As its name suggests, wind-relieving pose (*pavanmuktasana*) releases gas from the digestive system. To practice, lie on the back and clasp the legs to the chest, knees together. Make several clockwise circles with the knees, and then go the other direction. This helps massage the colon. The static version of the pose is also said to help dyspepsia and relieve acid reflux.

Spinal twists help push waste out of the body. Just be sure to twist to the right first (twisting to the right compresses the ascending colon, while twisting left compresses the descending colon). To practice *sukha ardha matsyendrasana* (easy seated half-twist), sit on a mat with the legs in front of you. Place the right foot on the outside of the left knee, with the foot flat on the mat. Place the right hand behind you. Clasp the right knee with the left arm, lift the chest, and twist to the right. Hold for five to 20 breaths while breathing into the belly. Then switch sides. This pose is also said to stimulate the pancreas, liver, spleen, kidneys, and stomach.

Other poses helpful for digestion include deep forward folds, *mayurasana* (peacock pose) and on-the-belly poses such as cobra, *dhanurasana* (bow), and *salabasana* (locust). Practices such as *kapalabhati* (shining skull breathing) and *agnisara kriya* (fire essence cleansing) also help but should be learned directly from a qualified teacher.

Try to avoid being too rigid in your practice. If you always do the same sequence, mix things up now and then. Try a new pose, or bind your hands or cross your legs in a different way from time to time.

Diet

Eat at the same time each day. Take your largest meal at lunch, and avoid heavy food after 8 p.m. (see "Eat Like a Yogi").

Start the day with a spoonful of ghee or flax oil, and follow it up with a glass of hot water with lemon or lime (to stimulate the digestive fire).

Digestion begins in the mouth. Chew each mouthful of food 25 times before swallowing, or until it is mushy. Avoid overeating. It takes about 20 minutes for the brain to get the message that the stomach is full. By eating slowly, you will feel full before your meal ends.

Avoid meat, fish, poultry, eggs, and cheese, which are difficult to digest, and stay away from frozen, processed, or leftover food for the same reason. Steer clear of white flour and dry foods such as crackers, pastries, and chips. Cold foods such as salads and ice cream and cold drinks with ice can "freeze" or slow down the digestive process. Avoid alcohol and limit sweets, which steal the B vitamins needed for the intestines to function.

Drink at least eight glasses of water per day, but also consume a lot of ghee or high-quality oils, such as olive oil, which lubricate the system. Try not to drink water with meals "as it dilutes the gastric juices essential for proper digestion," according to *Diet Cure for Common Ailments* by Dr. H. K. Bakhru. Instead, he recommends drinking water a half hour before eating or an hour after eating. Coffee and strong tea won't help, although they may seem to have an effect in the short term (caffeine is a diuretic that can remove water needed by the colon to process stool). Replace with fresh ginger tea.

Work more warm, moist, and naturally sweet foods into your diet. Whole, natural vegetables, grains, and legumes are best. Fruit should be eaten alone and on an empty stomach for maximum absorption. Avoid bananas, which can bind, and replace them with pineapple, a natural laxative that's also good for nausea. Grapes, pears, peaches, and plums are also recommended.

For breakfast, have something warm, moist, and sweet. I eat oatmeal cooked with raisins that have been soaked for 20 minutes. For lunch, try kitchari (an easy-to-digest stew of moong beans and rice) cooked with cumin and turmeric (see "Kitchari, Yoga's Wonder Food"). A wonderful snack or light supper is sweet potatoes slathered with ghee or olive oil.

Lifestyle

The body likes a routine. Get up and go to bed at the same time each day. When you feel the urge to defecate, give in to it as soon as possible. Holding the stool only leads to more problems down the road.

Many years ago, a colonic irrigationist suggested I take a daily probiotic, called Primal Defense Ultra. After taking it, my bowels moved better, and I got sick far less often. The ayurvedic herb mixture called triphala can have a similar effect; the recommended dose is 1/2 to one teaspoon at night, taken in hot water.

Exercise every day. Dr. Bahkru recommends going for brisk walks that last at least 45 minutes. Try to do this outside, in nature—the great healer—especially near water. As Swami Sivananda said, "The law of nature operates in the upkeep of the health of man."

Conclusion

Controlling constipation requires effort and change. But once your bowels move better, you may find that you have more energy and fall ill far less often.

I recommend choosing a few techniques that resonate with you. After integrating them into your routine, add a few more. Be patient, and think of it as part of your *sadhana* (practice). As the *Yoga Sutras* says, "practice becomes well-grounded when continued with reverent devotion and without interruption over a long period of time."

Going Head-to-Head with Headaches

"I will not be as those who spend the day in complaining of headache, and the night in drinking the wine that gives it."
—Goethe

I got my first headache when I was eight years old. The pain over my right eye was so excruciating I could barely get out of bed.

Fast-forward three decades to my first week studying Ashtanga yoga with the Jois family in Mysore, India. I had a migraine so intense that I vomited (and did not go to class). When the headache finally wore off I visited a doctor, who could not find a cause and sent me to an eye specialist. My eyes were fine. But he speculated that the migraine was probably caused by a banana and chocolate frozen smoothie I'd consumed, which contained three known migraine triggers (green banana, chocolate, and yogurt) as well as being a frozen food (a fourth trigger).

I've suffered from many, many headaches over the years—those two were the worst—and have learned that how I manage them can depend on the type of headache. (For years I suffered from sinus headaches but got no relief because I was trying to treat them as tension headaches.) In general, migraines can include nausea and vision changes; sinus headaches are focused behind the forehead or cheekbones; cluster headaches are centered in and around one eye (like the one I had as a child), and tension headaches, the most common type, feature constant pain—especially at the temples or back of the head. (If a headache lasts more than two days or is accompanied by a fever, stiff neck, blurred vision, difficulty with coordination or speech, forgetfulness, or weakness in the limbs, see a doctor.)

Regardless of type, many headaches have their source in emotional stress, poor diet, and/or tension in the neck and shoulders. Here are some techniques that have worked for me and for others.

Asana (yoga postures)

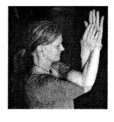

Simple shoulder rolls as well as shoulder and neck stretches such as *gomukasana* (cow face) and *garudasana* (eagle) may be practiced while seated at a desk. For garudasana place your right elbow on top of the left, in the crook of the elbow. Bend the elbows so that the forearms are perpendicular to the floor. Bring the hands together and slowly move the elbows up and down and sideways. Continue for several breaths and repeat on the other side.

For gomukasana, raise the right arm toward the ceiling, next to the ear. Bend the elbow and walk the hand down the back towards the shoulder blades. Bring the left arm straight out to the side; bend the elbow, and walk the hand up the back with the palm facing out. If possible, clasp hands. Press the hands into your back and gently move your elbows back behind you. Keep the head straight. Hold for several deep breaths and repeat on the other side.

Moving from sphinx to cobra relieves tension in the back, neck, and shoulders. Lie on the belly with the left ankle crossed over the right ankle. Place the elbows directly beneath the shoulders, so that the upper arms are vertical and the forearms are on the mat, parallel to each other. Move the shoulders toward the buttocks. After several breaths, lift the elbows off the floor until you are in cobra pose. Retract the chin and gaze straight ahead. After several breaths, slowly lower the elbows. Repeat with the ankles crossed the other way. Then relax in child's pose with your arms extended in front of you, palms up.

My sinus headaches have been relieved by backbends such as cobra, *dhanurasana* (bow) and *urdvha danurasana* (upward-facing bow), and headstand, while sun salutations and shoulderstand can make the throbbing worse.

In his seminal 1966 book *Light on Yoga*, for relieving headaches, BKS Iyengar recommended practicing supported headstand and shoulderstand for 10 minutes each, as well as plow for five minutes, *pascimottanasana* (seated forward bend) for five minutes (try it with your head on a pillow), and *uttanasana* (standing forward bend) for three minutes. (Headstand and shoulderstand should be avoided by those with neck, eye, heart, or blood pressure problems.)

A student once told me that a headache he'd had for a month finally disappeared when he opened his mouth wide to yawn. He'd inadvertently done *simhasana* (lion pose), which reduces tension and stress in the jaw, throat, neck, and face. To practice, sit on a chair or kneel on the floor. Press the palms into the thighs with the fingers spread wide apart. Inhale and close the eyes. While exhaling, pop the eyes open and gaze between the eyebrows while sticking out the tongue toward the chin and making a "Haaa" sound. Repeat four times.

Restorative poses—particularly those detailed in Judith Lasater's 1995 book *Relax and Renew: Restful Yoga for Stressful Times*—calm the nerves and relax the body. My favorite is her supported bridge pose: Lie on two bolsters placed end-to-end, with the feet on the bolster and the head and shoulders on the floor (a neck roll may be placed at the base of the neck, and the eyes and temples may be tightly wrapped in a cloth or covered with an eye pillow). Hold for five to 15 minutes, and come out of the pose slowly.

The most important pose for headache is *savasana* (corpse pose). I once led a patient undergoing long-term cancer treatment through savasana in her hospital room. Afterward she said she did not feel the headache she'd been suffering from for two weeks. Try it with a neck roll at the base of the skull, a bolster behind the knees, and an eye pillow or headache band covering the eyes. Stay for at least seven minutes.

Other yoga practices

Deep breathing into the belly reduces stress and tension in the neck and shoulders, while shallow breathing can cause them. A few rounds of *kapalabhati* (shining skull breathing) followed by 10 to 12 minutes of *anuloma vioma* (alternate nostril breathing) without retention of the breath can also minimize headaches; these last two practices should be learned directly from a qualified teacher.

My sinus headaches all but disappeared once I learned to use the neti pot at Sri Dharma Mittra's 2007 teacher training; now I do it every morning. Reducing meat, wheat, and dairy consumption will also help clear the sinuses.

I got a terrible headache between sessions at a retreat led by Dharma Mittra in 2010 in Mexico; it went away as soon as we did a practice in our lineage called sound breathing. Simply repeating Om for ten minutes (with a gap to breathe in between each utterance) can reduce head pain. I've also had headaches disappear while doing *japa* (meditative repetition of a mantra or divine name) and *kirtan* (call-and-response chanting).

Prevention: diet and lifestyle

Drink plenty of water; sometimes headaches are caused by simple dehydration (if you're drinking enough, your urine will be clear or very pale in color, not bright yellow).

Do not strain the neck in poses such as cobra, warrior I, and upward-facing dog. Instead, look straight ahead or down in these poses.

Headache triggers can vary from person to person. For example, I've found that medjool dates can trigger a headache (as will altitude and air travel). Common triggers include chocolate, bananas, wine and other alcohol, monosodium glutamate (MSG), caffeine, cheese, ice cream, frozen drinks, nightshades (such as tomatoes, potatoes, and eggplant), and the nitrates used in processed meat. Other causes include overeating or undereating (see "Eat Like a Yogi").

Headaches can also be caused by menopause, eye strain, high blood pressure, allergies, infection, low blood sugar, poor diet, toxins in the body, anemia, constipation, insomnia, stress, and intense emotions—each of which has a different cure. (Remedies for these causes of headache can be found in Dr. H. K. Bakhru's *The Complete Handbook of Nature Cure*, enlarged 5th edition published in 2010.)

To reduce tension in the neck and shoulders, breathe deeply into the belly throughout the day. Keep the spine straight and the chin tucked in, even when working or using your phone (are you slumping as you read this?). Switch which shoulder your carry bags on. And support your neck with a proper pillow when you sleep (and avoid sleeping on your stomach).

Make time to relax. Walk in nature at least once a week. Take a weekly restorative yoga class. Get plenty of sleep and do not skip savasana when you practice yoga.

As Dr. Bakhru writes, "The best remedy to prevent headache is to build up physical resistance through proper nutrition, exercise and constructive thinking."

Part Five: Diet, Health, and Healing

{42}

Eight Ways to Reduce Anxiety

"Nature does not hurry, yet everything is accomplished."
—Lao Tzu

Stressed out? You're not alone. Anxiety has replaced depression as America's top mood disorder, affecting 40 million adults in the United States age 18 and older, or over 18% of the population, according to the Anxiety and Depression Association of America.

Many of us who suffer from anxiety don't necessarily have a disorder, since it's a natural reaction to stress. But when we get overstressed, our body moves from rest-and-digest mode under the control of the parasympathetic nervous system into the fight-or-flight response generated by the sympathetic nervous system. Being constantly in fight-or-flight mode can lead to sleep disorders, migraines, chronic pain, hypertension, and other problems.

The first and best remedy is to practice yoga, of course—and to not skip savasana (corpse pose).

Here are a few other tips that may improve your mood.

1. Put the phone down and ask yourself: Do I control my phone, or does it control me?

Being constantly bombarded by blasts, tweets, texts, emails, calls, likes, and swipes can make anyone a nervous wreck. I remember being on the retreat I lead in Belize one year, when the WiFi was spotty. After a few days offline, my phone started buzzing with texts from a student who was scheduled to sub one of my classes back home. The first SMS said she'd forgotten the address. The second text was more frantic; she was downtown and couldn't find the place. The third one said she'd found it, and they'd had a great class. And I missed the entire drama—and all of the stress that went with it.

So, consider putting your phone on airplane mode for a few hours a few times a week, and switch off your news notifications so that you're not bombarded with nonstop crises. If you're receiving unwanted texts from someone, turn off notifications from their number. And switch off your phone at night so you can get some sleep.

2. Take 10 deep breaths. Then do it again. And again. And again.

Breathing deeply into the abdomen (not chest) is a quick and effective way to calm your mind, slow your thoughts, and reduce your stress level. Breathing through the nose is more efficient than breathing through the mouth, and belly breathing pulls more energy into your body and lets more tension out. You can teach yourself how to breathe deeply on a regular basis—something we all did as infants—by setting your cell phone alarm to go off several times a day; each time it does, take 10 deep breaths (do not hit the snooze button!). (For more, see "Change Your Breathing, Change Your Life.")

3. Eat less meat. Or give it up entirely.

Angry or fearful? My guru, Sri Dharma Mittra, says that when animals are slaughtered, they experience anger and fear and release adrenaline; when we eat their meat, we ingest those same emotions. He once had a student who complained that he had been meditating regularly for years but wasn't making any progress. Dharma asked him what he did for a living. He said he was a butcher. "If you eat too much spicy or animal-based food, you'll never be able to concentrate on anything," Sri Dharma says. "Without the ethical rules [of yoga], you're just wasting your time. It's like digging your own grave, and it causes lots of pain and delusion and disappointment."

4. Come into the present. Let the past and future go for just a little while.

Much of our stress comes from fears about the future or from ruminating on something that happened in the past. Oakland,

California–based meditation and yoga philosophy teacher Jim Gilman has a great trick for coming into the present moment: Pay attention to your breathing. Continue to connect with your breath while rubbing two fingers together. At the same time, listen to the sounds in the room. Doing these three things at once pulls you out of your reverie and brings you immediately into the present moment.

5. Forgive and apologize. Even if you're right.

Is it better to be right, or stress free? So much unnecessary anxiety comes from holding grudges and refusing to forgive or apologize. If someone has wronged you, holding on to it will only make you feel worse. Christian theologian Lewis B. Smedes said, "To forgive is to set a prisoner free and discover that the prisoner was you."

There are many ways to express forgiveness. It can be done in person, on the phone, in a thoughtful email, or in a handwritten letter. It can also be done mentally, if the person is no longer around or still poses a threat to you.

Sometimes we realize we have caused harm and need to ask forgiveness, which can be done in much the same way. Just keep it simple and straightforward: name exactly what you are sorry for, express your regret at causing harm, and do not make excuses for your behavior. And don't forget to forgive yourself, too.

6. Spend time in nature at least once a week. No excuses.

One of the greatest antidotes to anxiety and depression is spending time in nature, whether it be a forest preserve, a city park, a yard, or a simple walk around the block.

"People have been discussing their profound experiences in nature for the last several hundred years—from Thoreau to John Muir to many other writers," researcher David Strayer of the University of Utah told Greater Good Magazine reporter Jill Suttie in 2016, "Now we are seeing changes in the brain and changes in the body that suggest we are physically and mentally more healthy when we are interacting with nature."

Being in nature can reduce blood pressure, muscle tension, and the production of stress hormones. In a 2014 study researchers in Finland found that urban dwellers who strolled for as little as 20 minutes through an urban park or woodland reported significantly more stress relief than those who strolled in a city center, according to ScienceDirect.com.

7. Follow your heart. Not your head.

Sometimes, the conflict between our mind and intuition causes untold amounts of low-level stress, and we end up living a life that feels comfortable but inauthentic. So, is there something you know in your heart that you should be doing, but you've been avoiding or putting off? Is there something you'd dearly love to try, but your mind has been talking you out of it?

Is there a way you can begin to weave this thing into your life—or work towards it—even if it's for as little as 10 minutes a day? Meditate on it, and see what comes up.

As Elizabeth Gilbert wrote in her 2015 book, *Big Magic: Creative Living Beyond Fear*, "The universe buries strange jewels deep within us all, and then stands back to see if we can find them."

8. Help others. And ask for help when you need it.

We are not in this alone, and the easiest way to remember this is by helping others, whether it's formally through volunteering, or informally, like helping someone you encounter on the street carry their groceries. In addition to being a yoga practice, *Karma* yoga (yoga of action) or *seva* (selfless service) offers a way to get out of your head, reduce anxiety, and connect with others (see "Make an Offering: *Karma* Yoga")

On the flipside, I recently got over my aversion to asking for help and learned that receiving help has the same result as helping others; it makes me feel connected and empowered. Asking for help can foster personal growth, as it requires a certain amount of humility. Remember, life is a group effort, and none of us can "do it all" on our own.

Om Tat Sat

About the Author

Kali Om has taught yoga since 1998 to a wide range of students at a variety of settings, which in addition to yoga studios, include a hospital cancer ward, a cruise ship, a city park, an airport gate, an exclusive health club, a nursing home, and at the end of a Caribbean pier. She has taught full-time since 2004.

She is registered beyond the highest level (E-RYT 500) of the Yoga Alliance's standards and has a master's degree in journalism. She is a columnist and cartoonist for *Yoga Chicago* magazine and serves as co-chair of the Vivekananda East-West International Yoga Festival.

Her yoga studies include 200-, 500-, and 800-hour trainings with her guru, Sri Dharma Mittra. Between 2002 and 2008 she made five trips to India to study Ashtanga Vinyasa yoga with Pattabhi Jois and his family. In addition, she is certified to teach pranayama (breathwork), meditation, Hormone Yoga Therapy for Menopause, prenatal yoga, Yoga Nidra, psychic development, gentle/restorative yoga, Rocket Yoga, yoga for seniors, and yoga therapeutics. She specializes in yoga for back problems and yoga for anxiety, depression, and stress. She leads workshops, teacher trainings, and retreats in the U.S. and abroad. She teaches as an offering to her guru.

Studying Yoga with Kali

Kali Om offers ongoing yoga classes and leads yoga vacations, satsangs (spiritual gatherings), and teacher trainings. She also teaches weekend workshops and private lessons in person and via Skype and video chat, which are open to students and teachers at all levels. For her teaching schedule, or to invite her to give classes, workshops or retreats at your venue, please visit www.yogikaliom.com.